A First Notebook of HEAD INJURY

A First Notebook of
HEAD INJURY

Second Edition

KENNETH G. JAMIESON
M.D., M.S. (Melb.), F.R.A.C.S., F.A.C.S.
Senior Visiting Neurosurgeon, Royal Brisbane Hospital, and Royal Children's Hospital, Brisbane; Lecturer in Neurosurgery, University of Queensland

BUTTERWORTHS
LONDON - BOSTON
Sydney - Wellington - Durban - Toronto

The Butterworth Group

United Kingdom	**Butterworth & Co (Publishers) Ltd** London: 88 Kingsway, WC2B 6AB
Australia	**Butterworths Pty Ltd** Sydney: 586 Pacific Highway, Chatswood, NSW 2067 Also at Melbourne, Brisbane, Adelaide and Perth
Canada	**Butterworth & Co (Canada) Ltd** Toronto: 2265 Midland Avenue, Scarborough, Ontario, M1P 4S1
New Zealand	**Butterworths of New Zealand Ltd** Wellington: T & W Young Building, 77–85 Customhouse Quay, 1 CPO Box 472
South Africa	**Butterworth & Co (South Africa) (Pty) Ltd** Durban: 152–154 Gale Street
USA	**Butterworth (Publishers) Inc** Boston: 10 Tower Office Park, Woburn, Mass. 01801

First published 1965, by Jacaranda Press Pty Ltd
73 Elizabeth Street, Brisbane
Second edition 1971, by Butterworth & Co. (Publishers) Ltd
Reprinted 1976
Reprinted 1978
Reprinted 1979

Suggested U.D.C. Number 616–001: 611·91
Suggested additional numbers 617·51

ISBN 0 407 17350 1

Printed in Great Britain by offset lithography
by Billing & Sons Ltd, Guildford, London and Worcester

To the skill and devotion
of every nurse who accepts her important responsibility
for the care of patients with Head Injury
this book is dedicated

Contents

PART IV: PHYSIOLOGY AND NURSING CARE

PART V

Preface to the Second Edition

Compiled originally for the use of local medical students and practitioners and of nurses in the Australian environment, this book has found a gratifyingly wider readership and a demand that warranted a second edition.

The basic treatment of head injury is to a great extent unchanged. Recent researches, though increasing our understanding of many matters, have not yet made practical impact on the management of such injuries.

A section on the temporal lobes and memory disturbance and sources of further reading have been added for this edition. Additional notes on respiration and electrolyte balance are provided also. For increasing appreciation of these subjects I am indebted to our senior anaesthetist, Dr. Tess Brophy, whose continuing interest in individual patient care has been of service to so many of our patients.

In parallel with the demand for better clinical care, which is the subject of this work, is an increasingly urgent need for surgeons to accept the responsibilities of prevention of trauma. Experience indicates that head injuries are becoming progressively more severe as the human body is subjected to ever more violent impact, especially on the roads. Unless this energy expenditure on the head can be mitigated, the future is one of increasing inefficacy of our available methods of treatment.

Brisbane, February 1971 KENNETH G. JAMIESON

Preface to the First Edition

There is scarcely need to stress the importance of head injury to anyone who scans the daily newspapers. Road accident is the commonest cause of death of young people, and head injury claims most of the victims. To these may be added those from accident at sport, at work and at home to produce a frightening total. Among the survivors, physical and mental handicaps represent major disasters, quite apart from the social and economic loss to the community.

Much of this toll is irreducible unless the accidents can be prevented but adequate surgical care will alleviate the position. Especially in our country, Australia, where distances are great, accident victims in small agricultural communities may be separated by hundreds of miles from a specialist surgeon, while neurosurgical aid may be more than a thousand miles away. Thus the necessity for every doctor to have a clear concept of the nature of these injuries and ability to treat them. Thus also the need to present these matters in clear form, even at the expense of dogmatism, and without that mystery with which the specialist tends to surround his subject.

The style of this notebook is selected for that great body of medical illiterates who, like the author, learn more geography from travel books than from factual tones, and prefer murder stories to formal prose at the end of the day. The student who yawns after a few pages of a textbook will read avidly from a paperback. It seems extraordinary that what we really want to read should be made so unreadable and indigestable that its message is lost. To the fortunate remaining literates, my apologies.

What is here set out represents the discipline adopted in the Brisbane Hospital and the Brisbane Children's Hospital. It is that followed also at the Princess Alexandra Hospital, Brisbane, where I assist the Surgical Staff with the care of patients with head injury.

All of the observations and recommendations made are based upon our daily practice, but no special claim is made here to originality in any of them. The paucity of literature references to the work of others represents neither unconsciousness of it, nor ingratitude for the opportunity of benefiting from it.

A few particular acknowledgements are my privilege.

Mr. Reginald Hooper of Melbourne placed my interest in head injuries on sound foundations, and should any part of what follows show that I have built ill on these, he is not to blame. He is assured my lasting gratitude and enduring respect, and continuing endeavour to emulate his understanding and ability.

My hospital staff colleagues have assisted me with co-operation and encouragement, while the resident and nursing staffs are responsible for much of what success we can claim. Dr. J.D.N. Yelland, first my Registrar and now my valued colleague, shares ably and willingly the obligations of a head injury service, while all members of our Neurosurgical Unit, and the Queensland Government Pathologist, Dr. John Tonge, are my creditors.

Preparation of such a work as this involves careful review of one's own clinical experience. This could not have been achieved without the aid of a grant to our neurosurgical unit from the Margaret Hart Martin Bequest for Brain and Cancer Research in the University of Queensland, the assistance of which is gratefully recorded.

It is a pleasure to acknowledge the valuable criticism of this work offered by Dr. D.A. Henderson and Dr. J.M. Sutherland, and the enthusiastic and accurate work of Mrs P. Cremonesi and Miss D. Wilson in preparing the manuscript.

Most of all I am in debt to the many patients who have been the basis of this book. Would that I had been able to discharge my debt to a greater proportion of them.

Brisbane, May 1964 KENNETH G. JAMIESON

Part I
The Coverings

It is said that one cannot judge a book by its cover, but which of us does not peruse the title on the cover as a clue to the contents?

Just as surely does the bruise on the scalp, or other physical sign of trauma, give a clue to the state of the brain. Unless one knows the nature and mechanism of the injury, which the coverings so often depict, one knows little of value to the patient.

In no other branch of surgery is it fashionable to ignore the site of trauma, seeking no local signs, and to be preoccupied with function at a distance. But of head injury we are told, 'It is the brain that counts, not scalp and skull' – so the novice turns to the knee jerks and misses his vital clues.

Examine the cover first and you may know what can be expected within. Since the coverings are usually injured, let us start where we should and proceed inward.

1—Scalp Injuries

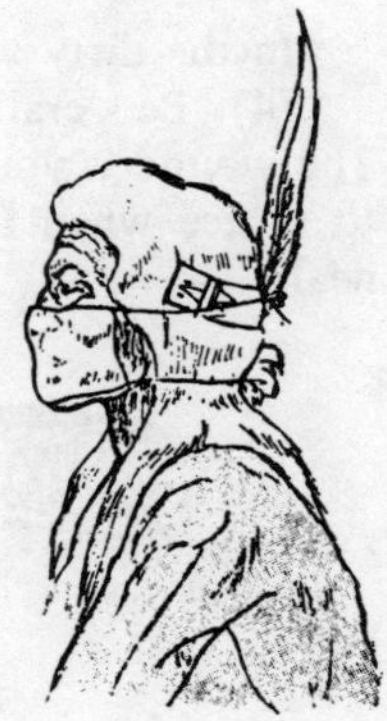

Scalp hunting is an old occupation, but it becomes time-honoured only if one obeys the rules of the game.

Be a scalp hunter! Search for the bruise or the laceration, the small abrasion (often not seen until after shaving) or the haematoma. These may be the only indications as to the site of trauma and the site for exploration.

Stick to the rules! The surgeon who collects scalps must shave them, cleanse them, prepare them, and so suture or dress them that they will heal without mischance. Infection of the scalp is perilous, readily communicated by emissary veins to the brain itself. Osteomyelitis, extradural and subdural abscess, cortical thrombophlebitis and brain abscess may pronounce the death penalty for neglect of even a small wound. Will it occur from your practice? So back to first principles in wound toilet and care.

(1) Shave widely and cleanse thoroughly.

(2) Suture without tension.

Over intact surrounding pericranium, which can granulate safely or be grafted, you may

Relax or relieve or advance as you will
As long as you cover the wound.

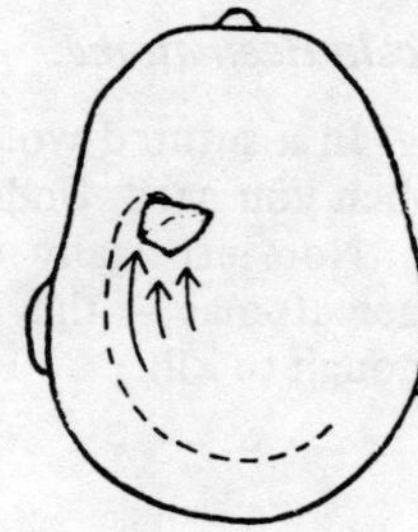

(3) Appose all layers, and allow the wound to heal.

The most important layer is the galea aponeurotica, which tends to retract and gape. Unless it is reconstituted, a thin weak scar may result, and tension on the skin may endanger the blood supply in the superficial vascular layer of scalp, leading to wound breakdown. Haemostasis is most readily achieved by suturing the galea. Sew it separately, with inverted sutures, in the clean wound.

In the dirty wound, don't bury silk, but use the 'safety-pin' stitch.

(4) Be a craftsman.

The wound is your signature. If it is careless, the patient will have cause to notice when he consults his mirror or uses his comb. Neat wounds heal.

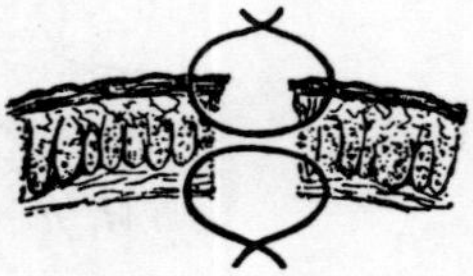

2 LAYERS

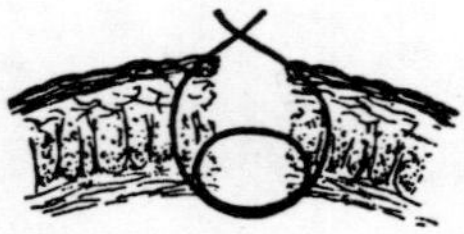

SAFETY-PIN STITCH

Problem Corner

Scalp Loss

Do not throw away viable scalp. Be sparing with excision of skin edges. Test the mobility of the scalp before you excise the wound to be sure you can close it.

If scalp is lost over the wound, rotate or undercut and advance neighbouring scalp to cover it, and graft the pericranium of the donor site.

If bone edge is exposed and not capable of cover, excise it and let dura granulate.

If a raw bone area is exposed and incapable of cover, excise it or drill the outer table and allow diploe to granulate.

Scalp Haematoma

In a sutured wound, clots get infection for lack of a drain. Use one when you need. Under closed scalp, aspirate the haematoma if large.

Note especially that small infants may exsanguinate into subgaleal haematomas – this blood loss without external haemorrhage may be enough to kill.

2—Fractures

'. . . . The time has been
That, when the brains were out, the man would die,
And there an end; but now they rise again . . . .'
Macbeth, Act III, Scene IV

'Fractured skull' is a layman's terminology for head injury, and his measure of its severity. Medico-legally, radiological proof of fracture may be of great moment, but the clinical significance of fracture is different. In the surgeon's view, the presence, site and type of fracture connote in some measure both the degree of violence and the likely complications of a head injury.

Certain groups require discussion.

LINEAR FRACTURES

Radiology provides neither the only nor the best evidence of fracture in all cases.

Examine the head!

Likely Sites of Fracture

Fractures tend not to cross bony buttresses, such as glabella, frontal and parietal eminences, petrous mass and occipital protuberance. Fractures tend to cross points of weakness – frontal sinuses and orbital roof, parietal and occipital squama.

From the site and direction of the blow on the scalp one can predict the likely fracture line.

Frontal

A blow over the glabella may cause shattering of the ethmoid sinuses and roof of the nose.

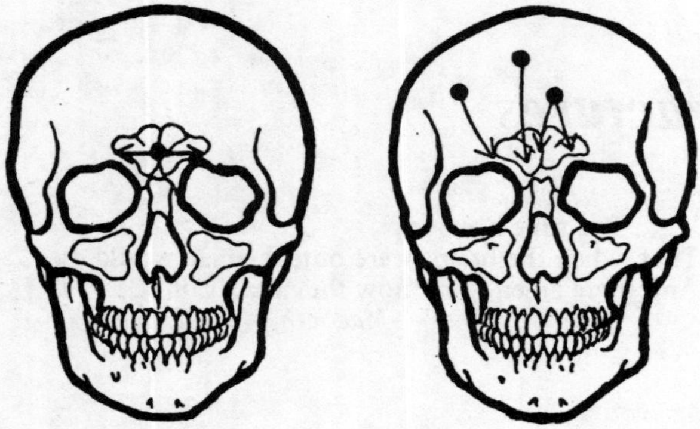

Blows higher on the forehead tend to cause fractures which cross the frontal sinus into the roof of the orbit. On some occasions they may traverse the optic foramen, especially when the blow is on the frontal eminence.

Lateral

A blow anywhere between or below the frontal and parietal eminences may cause a fracture which runs vertically or obliquely across the thin temporal squama to the floor of the middle, or sometimes the anterior, cranial fossa.

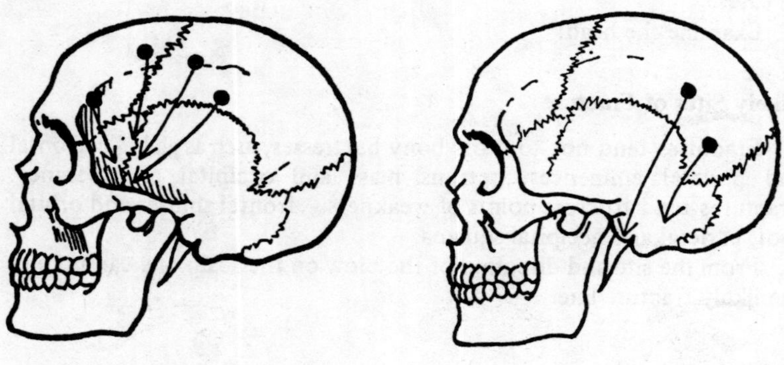

From the parietal eminence, fractures tend to run through the ear, while from behind it they run to the region of the mastoid.

Occipital

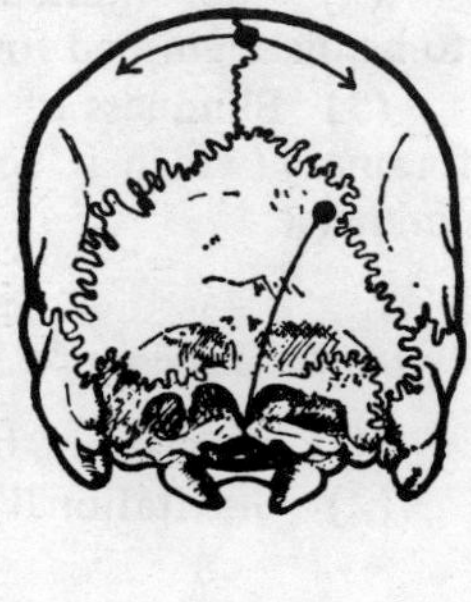

Blows on the occiput tend to cause fractures which descend vertically through the thin occipital squama to the foramen magnum.

Vertical

Blows high on the vertex tend to produce fractures which cross the midline, sometimes following suture lines.

Physical Signs of Fracture

With experience one's predictions become more accurate, but to them may be added physical signs of fracture at various sites.

Roof of Nose and Accessory Nasal Sinuses

(1) Escape of air into the tissues – subcutaneous emphysema on forehead.

(2) Escape of intracranial content through the nose – cerebrospinal fluid rhinorrhoea, or escape of brain tissue.

(3) X-ray evidence of air within the skull – either within the ventricles, or in the region of the chiasm in the brow-up lateral view.

Orbits, Including Zygoma

(1) Orbital haematoma, limited by attachments of the orbital fascia – to be distinguished from the common black eye with ecchymoses over eyebrow, nose and malar.

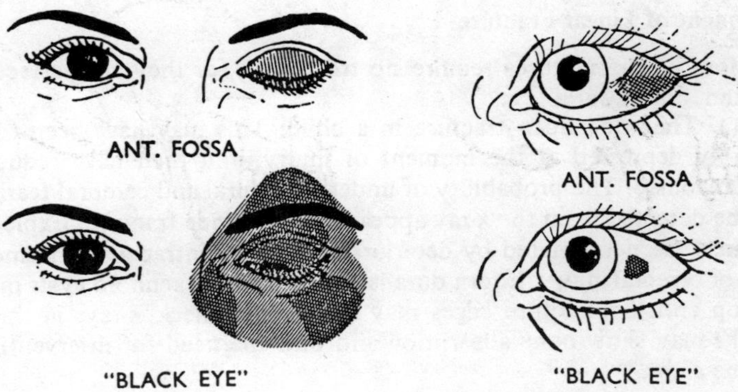

(2) Subconjunctival haematoma without visible posterior margin – to be distinguished form the local contusion of direct violence.

(3) Blindness of one eye, sometimes, if fracture involves the optic foramen (which it commonly skirts) from a blow usually on frontal eminence.

Temporal Squama or Sphenoid Wing

(1) Haematoma beneath temporal fascia – the classical 'bogginess'.
(2) Gravitational haematoma staining behind the ear.

Petrous Temporal

(1) Deafness in one ear.
(2) Facial nerve paralysis.
(3) Cerebrospinal fluid otorrhoea.

Posterior Fossa

Haematoma beneath suboccipital muscles, if trauma above them.

Anywhere

Subperiosteal haematoma is suggestive.

Do not confuse its edge, which may be dented by the thumbnail, with depressed fracture.

If you know where the fracture is, then be forewarned of the likely complications – what vessels, what nerves, what other structure may be damaged.

Treatment of Linear Fracture

Most linear fractures require no treatment, for they are perfectly splinted, but beware:

(1) The wide open fracture in a child. This may have been considerably depressed at the moment of injury, and then have reduced spontaneously. The probability of underlying dural and cerebral tearing may be detected from the x-ray appearance of a wide fracture. Exploration may be necessitated by deterioration due to intracranial haemorrhage or cerebral injury. If torn dura is not repaired, arachnoid cysts may develop and the fracture edges may be eroded. Check x-rays in three months may show bone absorption and thus the need for intervention in some cases.

(2) Compound linear fracture – be more meticulous than ever with that scalp!

(3) Fracture through accessory nasal sinuses or nose, especially in the presence of *cerebrospinal fluid rhinorrhoea.*

If you are in doubt as to whether fluid escaping from the nose is cerebrospinal fluid, collect some and test it for sugar.

The patient with cerebrospinal fluid rhinorrhoea should be told not to blow his nose or attempt to suppress a sneeze. Nothing should be passed through the nostril – oxygen or suction catheters are to be avoided.

Broad spectrum antibiotics should be given to prevent the occurrence of meningitis.

If the rhinorrhoea stops, this may be due to plugging of a hole in the dura by a cerebral hernia. The nose is thus directly roofed by brain, and the stage is then indeed set for cerebral abscess or meningitis, as much as if the rhinorrhoea continued.

Careful oblique (and stereoscopic) x-rays of the orbital roofs may show wide open fractures. If so, or if rhinorrhoea recurs, repair of the floor of the anterior fossa is mandatory, and the patient is best transferred to neurosurgical care.

(The usual technique is exposure intradurally of the floor of the anterior fossa through a frontal osteoplastic flap – bilaterally if necessary – and covering of the defects with a sheet of fascia lata, pericranium or muscle).

(4) Fractures through the ear, especially in the presence of *cerebrospinal fluid otorrhoea.* This latter usually stops safely, but no aural manipulation or plugging should be entertained.

Leave the ear strictly alone, cover it with a clean pad, and give broad spectrum antibiotics.

If the leak continues, repair will be needed.

DEPRESSED FRACTURES

These fall into two groups.

Smooth 'Pond' Fracture

This is a simple in-buckling of the skull, which results from the obstetric forceps blade, the sacral promontory in precipitate labour, or a blow from a blunt object. Historically, it is a very old type of fracture, likely to have been caused by caveman wooing fair maiden with a club. The injury so sustained is likely to have been more innocent than the caveman's intentions.

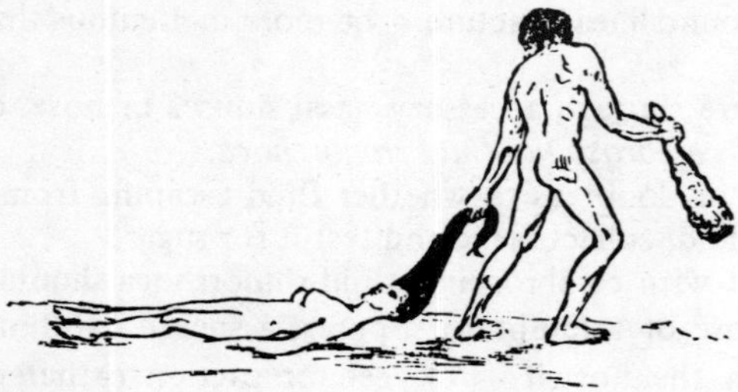

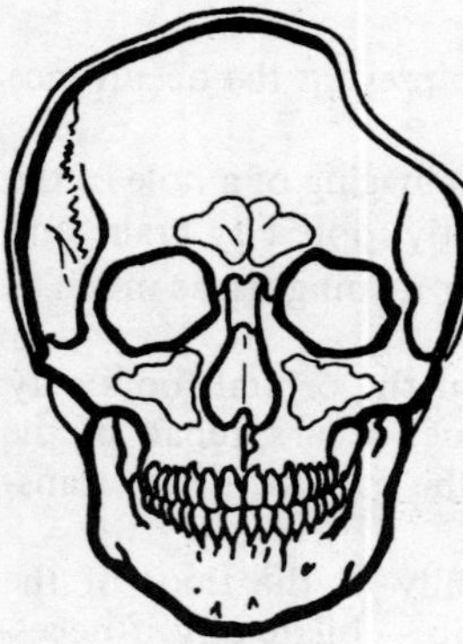

"POND"

The inner table does not fragment, the dura mater is not torn, and the brain is usually undamaged. All that is required is a burrhole at the edge, a lever under the depression, and elevation of the bone. In infants, do this if the depression is large, if signs of cerebral compression appear, if a suture is involved or for cosmetic reasons.

Many such fractures, caused at the moment of impact, spontaneously reduce. If x-ray shows a circular fracture line, this must have occurred.

Narrow 'Gutter' or Comminuted Depression

This is a very different lesion. The inner table is fragmented, dura mater and brain may be torn, and fragments of scalp or bone may be driven deep into the brain.

This is the result of a high velocity blow on a local area of the head, and a classic example is the vertical injury to the forehead when a tyre-lever slips. Projecting control-panel knobs, bonnet mascots and similar lethal instruments built into external and internal design of cars add to the toll when modern man woos fair maiden with a car!

These injuries require exploration–not simply elevation–for the dura and brain must be dealt with.

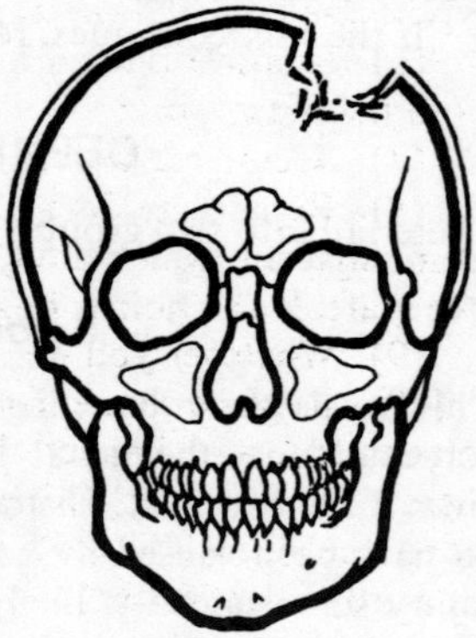

"GUTTER"

Operation for Compound Depressed Fracture

(1) If a laceration is present, enlarge it as you need; recurve the ends to give lateral exposure. (If the wound is dirty, skirt it with a flap of scalp, especially on the forehead to expose a supra-orbital fracture; this indirect approach often gives the best access.)

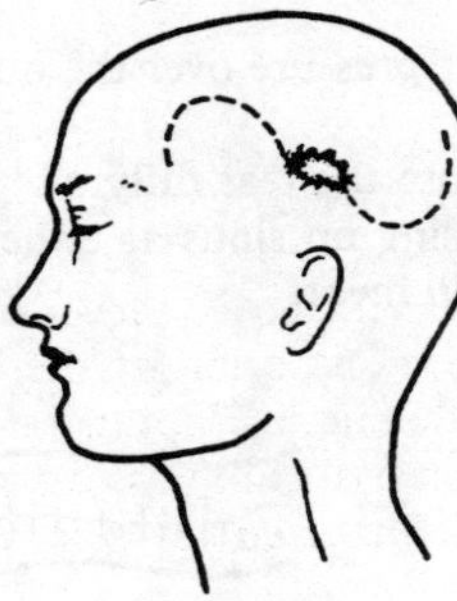

ENLARGE

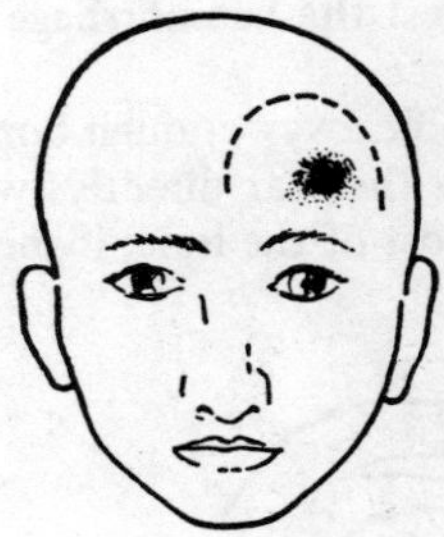

SKIRT

(2) Nibble away an over-riding edge of the outer table to uncover the edge of a depressed fragment and disimpact it. Reflect bone plates on pericranium, or discard them if devitalized and small.

(3) Slide out the deeper pieces rather than angulate them, for fear of increasing brain damage.

(4) Remove all pieces of inner table.

(5) Place guy sutures in the dural edges, and nibble away bone to expose the whole dural tear.

(6) Remove pulped brain by gentle suction, and all foreign bodies from the brain wound.

(7) Secure haemostasis, by diathermy, or ligation, or gelatin sponge.

(8) Repair the dura mater. If there is a defect, borrow pericranium from adjacent intact skull, rotating it on a pedicle or sewing it on as a free graft. If the hole is huge, use fascia lata.

(9) Whatever you do, repair the dura.

(10) Replace bone fragments if they have pericranial or muscle attachment, and impact them if they sit well (wire sutures may hold them). Do not fear to leave a large bone defect for later repair provided the dura is closed. Preserve the orbital margins if possible; they are hard to reconstruct.

The important step is to expose the whole dural tear and close it!

Be Warned

Should the fracture overlie a venous sinus – sagittal or transverse – the depressed bone fragments may so compress these structures that lacerations in them do not bleed.

Removal of the fragments may allow furious haemorrhage.

Repair of Venous Sinuses

(1) Arrest the haemorrhage by direct pressure over the hole in the sinus.

(2) Nibble away enough bone to expose the tear fully.

(3) Sew the tear directly, while pressing on sinus at either end or occluding most of the hole, if the edges will meet.

(4) If this solution is impracticable or fails, take a piece of temporal or suboccipital muscle, squash it flat, hold it over the tear and secure it under the mattress sutures through dura on either side.

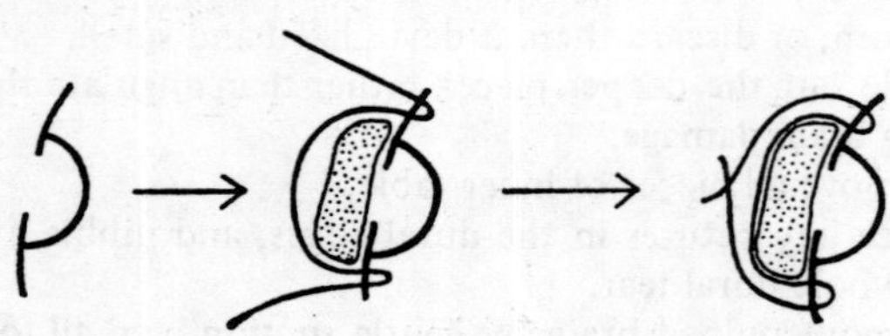

Be Optimistic!

Depressed fractures result from local violence, and absorb much of the energy of the blow. The impact on the brain as a whole is lessened. Considering the severity of the trauma, brain damage (except immediately beneath the fracture) is slight relative to what it might have been had the skull remained intact and the brain been accelerated or decelerated more violently. The prognosis depends often solely upon the neurological significance of the particular site of local brain damage.

Problem Corner

Skull Defects

A skull defect should be closed, at leisure, if:

(1) It is large and unsightly, for cosmetic reasons.

(2) The patient fears trauma over it, for psychological reasons.

(3) It pulsates, for the ventricle may expand towards it producing a ventricular diverticulum and local atrophy.

(4) It bulges when the patient stoops, and headache is suffered.

Large defects, especially in cosmetically significant areas such as the forehead, may require some experience and special facilities and materials (acrylic moulds or tantalum) for their closure.

Smaller defects are within the scope of any trained surgeon and do not need the expense and inconvenience of transport from remote centres to neurosurgical care. Ribgraft cranioplasty is then the method of choice (Appendix 2).

RECOMMENDED FURTHER READING

Dandy, W.E. (1926). 'Pneumocephalus'. *Archs Surg.,* Chicago **12**, 949

Gurdjian, E.S. and Webster, J.E. (1958). *Head Injuries: Mechanisms, Diagnosis and Management.* London: Churchill; Boston: Little Brown

Lewin, Walpole (1966). *The Management of Head Injuries.* London: Baillière, Tindall & Cassell

3—The Dura Mater and its Vessels

EXTRADURAL HAEMATOMA

One of the simplest concepts in surgery is that of a local bruise extending from skin through underlying tissues in the line of trauma. An extradural haematoma is simply a portion of such a bruise on the head, complicated only by the presence of a layer of bone between haematoma and skin. So slight a barrier should scarcely disturb any home handyman who has wielded brace and bit!

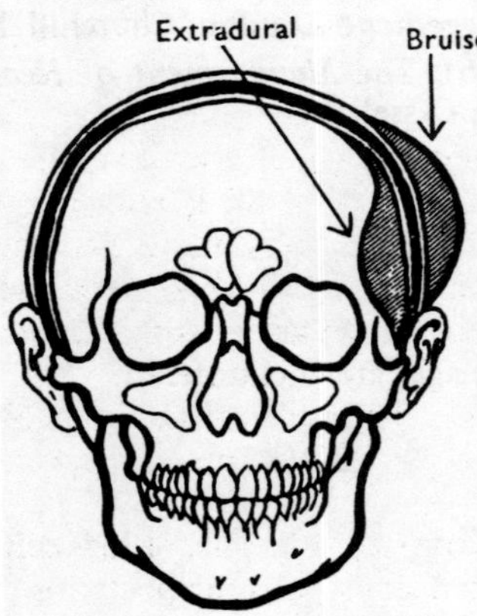

It is generally considered appropriate to write, after extradural haematoma, the explanation, 'Synonym: Middle Meningeal Haemorrhage'. This displays profound ignorance of the pathogenesis of the lesion, for the middle meningeal artery is involved in less than half the cases. Such confusion results in wrong selection of the site for exploration and accounts in part for the appalling mortality rate generally accepted.

Q. What is an extradural haematoma?

A. It is a collection of blood in the extradural space.

Q. What extradural space?

A. There is normally no extradural space for dura mater, which is the periosteum, is closely adherent to the skull.

Q. How is the space created?

A. It is produced by the injury itself in the first instance, and may be enlarged by further stripping of dura by active bleeding.

Consider the mechanism of the injury.

At the moment of impact, the elastic skull deforms. If this exceeds the limit of elasticity, linear or pond depressed fracture may occur. But in any case the skull moves relative to the dura beneath it, and the dura is stripped from the bone.

Thus an extradural space, empty, is created at the site of trauma, and only there.

At the same time a blood vessel may be injured. This may be a diploic vein in the course of a fracture (a subperiosteal haematoma is particularly suggestive of this) or a vessel in the dura mater. Note that, because of relative movement of bone on dura, even if fracturing does not occur, vessels – and especially the thin-walled veins – may be injured in the absence of fracture. Fracture is not essential to extradural haematoma.

The vessel injured depends upon the site of trauma.

Temporoparietal. A blow over the lateral convexity of the head may injure the middle meningeal artery, one of its major branches, or small terminal rami. However, it is more likely to be the thinner walled veins which groove the bone than the artery which is involved, although some brisk arterial haemorrhages are encountered.

Frontal. A blow over the forehead involves a different set of vessels, for here the blood supply of the dura is from the anterior ethmoidal artery.

Occipital. A blow over the occiput, or low behind the ear, may tear the transverse or sigmoid sinus; thus the posterior fossa haematoma.

Vertical. A blow on the vertex may cause haemorrhage from the sagittal sinus.

Thus the extradural haematoma arises from a locally injured vessel bleeding into a space created at the site of trauma.

The haematoma underlies the site of the blow (look for the bruise on the scalp), or the fracture line arising from it (you know where the latter is likely to run on clinical grounds, even if you have no x-rays).

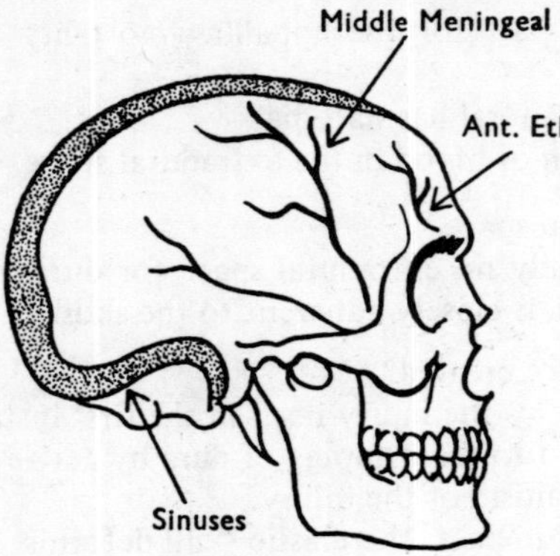

The haematoma cannot be contrecoup unless the skull has been grossly deformed. If it is bilateral, then trauma has been bilateral, or a midline structure (such as the sagittal sinus) has been injured.

In my own series of over 100 cases, the distribution has been roughly:

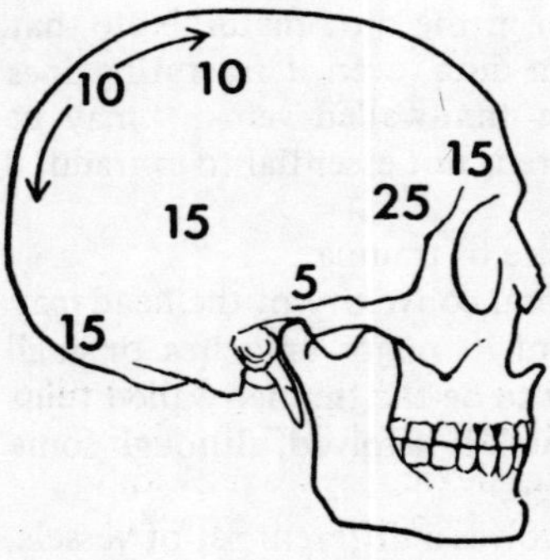

25 per cent anterior temporal.
15 per cent posterior temporal.
15 per cent anterior fossa.
15 per cent posterior fossa.
10 per cent high parietal.
10 per cent supratentorial from venous sinuses.
5 per cent exclusively floor of middle fossa.
5 per cent underlying depressed fractures

For present purposes it is convenient to defer until later discussion of the course of the lesion and the means of diagnosis. What concerns us now is the site of the lesion relative to surgery, and the operation to be done.

Drilling the Hole

The neurosurgeon may well be held responsible for the treatment of head injuries in major cities, but the urgency of extradural haemorrhage is well known. Especially in Australia, where distances are great, if operation is to be performed in time to save the life of the patient, the local practitioner must do it.

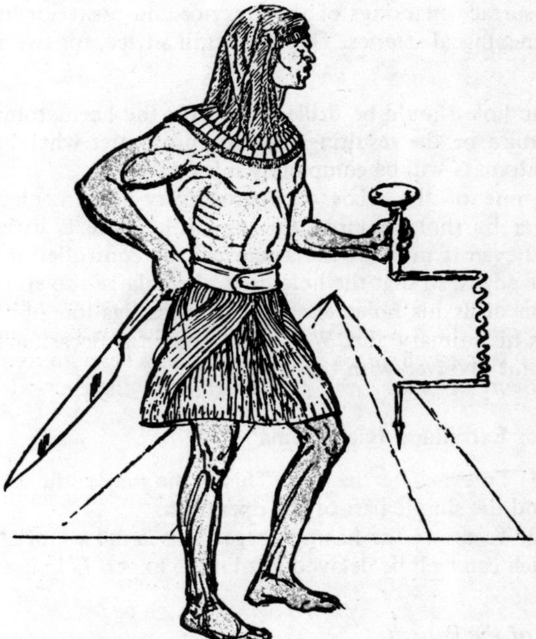

Who drills the hole?
Who's on the spot? –
There's no time for transfer!
The local Doc. must stand the shock
Of brace and bit and burr.
'Who, me?', you ask, 'But why, the task
Exceeds my slender skill'.
'Then shortly, friend the patient's end
Will come unless you drill'.

For as they built the pyramids
Egyptians drilled the skull.
In Mexico, as we now know,
The trepan ne'er grew dull.
The Incas in the Andes too
Found ventilation fine,
While ancient Babylonians
Could wield a neat trephine.

If they could do it, without your training, so can you.

Q. When?
A. As soon as the diagnosis is suspected
Q. Where?
A. At the site of trauma.

Ill Advice for the Innocent

This is the correct title for many standard textbook descriptions of where to drill the hole. The holes should be drilled, we are told, over the anatomical surface markings of the anterior and posterior branches of the middle meningeal arteries. This is most ill advice, for two reasons:

First, the hole should be drilled wherever the haematoma is, under the scalp bruise or the resulting fracture, no matter where. Otherwise many haematomata will be completely missed.

Second, one of the trials of neurosurgery is a meningeal artery bleeding in a burrhole, injured by the drill. There is little room to operate, and even if most of the artery can be controlled it often still bleeds at the edges, so that the hole has to be enlarged to stop it. So the neurosurgeon drills his holes elsewhere, unless ligation of the middle meningeal is his primary aim. Why then advise the occasional craniotomist to become involved with these vessels?

Operation for Extradural Haematoma

Object 1. To evacuate the clot. This is the major, the essential, the life-saving and the simple part of the operation.

Object 2. To arrest the haemorrhage. This is the minor and secondary step which can well be delayed until more expert help is available.

Preparation of the Patient

Two important factors require attention before any major neurosurgical operation:

The airway. – Respiration must be quite free throughout operation if further damage to the brain and troublesome bleeding are to be avoided. A pharyngeal airway may suffice for operation under local anaesthesia, but the drapes should be well supported so that they do not obstruct the airway or cause the patient to rebreathe from an enclosed space. If a pharyngeal airway is inadequate, pass an endotracheal tube, making sure that its end is in the trachea and not down into a bronchus.

Transfusion. – Much blood may be lost in the course of the operation. Start, or have someone else start, an intravenous infusion, and cross-match blood.

Evacuating the Clot

(1) Shave and prepare the scalp – if there is time. If the patient is in extremis, or deteriorating rapidly, the emergency is real. Time is all important, asepsis and routine can go by the board. Drill the hole unsterile and get out the clot. Then shave, prepare and sterilize, and start routinely to arrest bleeding. Give me the fertile quick, not the sterile dead!

(2) Mark your incision before draping the head – scratch it on the scalp while you are still orientated. It overlies the site of the blow, or skirts it flapwise if the scalp is contused and dirty.

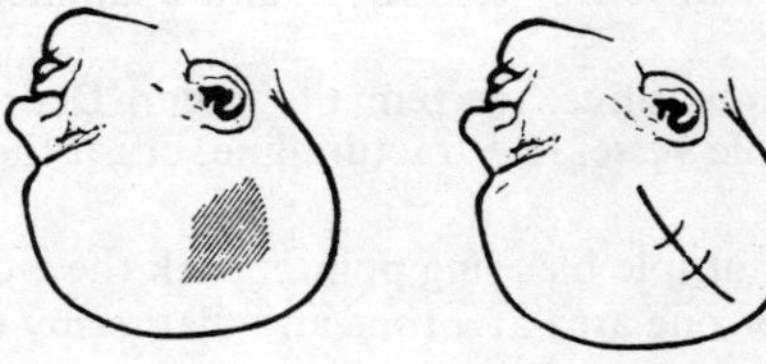

BRUISE INCISION MARKED

(3) Use a small cut, 2·5 cm will do. When you retract the edges, the stretch will provide haemostasis. If your site is wrong and you must look elsewhere, three stitches will close it. Cut straight to bone and elevate pericranium with scalp.

(4) Drill an inspection hole. If no haematoma is found, open the dura. If no subdural blood or fluid is found, see what the pressure is like. If it is high, you must look elsewhere. Close the scalp wound.

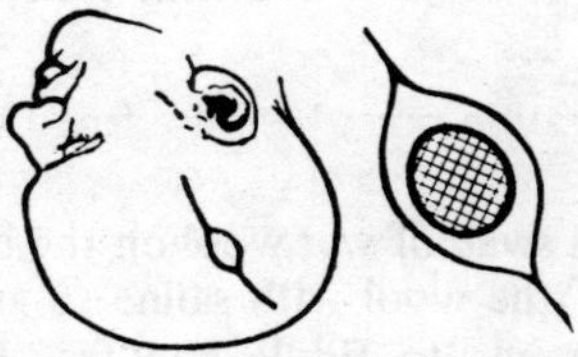

INSPECTION HOLE

(5) If haematoma is found, suck some out and, with a probe, discover in which direction the clot becomes thicker.

(6) Enlarge the scalp incision, straight or curved, to allow bone removal in the direction of deepening clot.

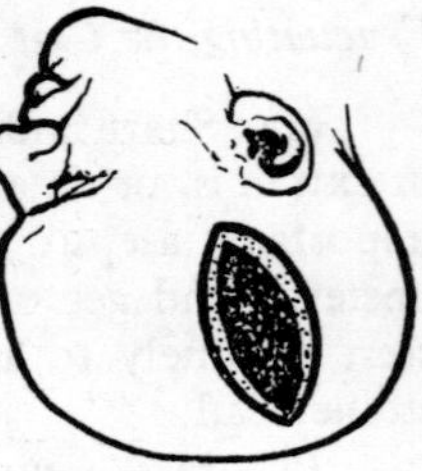

(7) Scrape back pericranium or muscle and nibble away bone to expose the clot.

(8) Wash away, suck away and scrape away clot. Use a dissector under bone edges. Make the hole in the skull big enough to see all the area involved.

At this stage, life has been saved

(9) Look for the bleeding point. It may be an artery; diathermy it, or under-run it with a suture and ligate it. (A matchstick in the foramen spinosum, beloved of textbooks and examiners, is a very rare necessity.)

It may be a venous sinus; see remarks under 'Depressed Fractures'.

It may be a diploic vessel in a fracture-line; crush the diploe, or pack it with bone wax.

There may be multiple bleeding points; pack the wound with pieces of wet wool. Uncover one area at a time and diathermy or under-run the the major points.

It may be from under bone edges; sew the dura to the pericranium hitching it against bone.

There may be multiple small oozes; cover with gelatin sponge or wool and take tea.

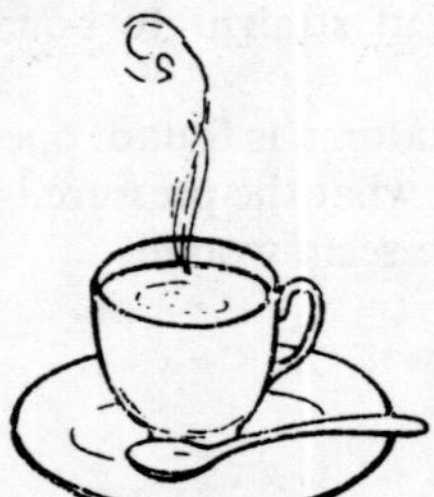

The best haemostat in the neurosurgical armamentarium is the time taken for tea

If all else fails, hold a swab of wet wool on the bleeding points until they stop, then wash off the wool with saline so as not to disturb the clot. (The neurosurgeon has to fiddle and fret like this; you have company!)

(10) Hitch dura to pericranium around the bone edges always; this prevents reaccumulation of clot.

(11) Open the dura; quite large amounts of cerebrospinal fluid, more or less bloodstained, are sometimes found.

(12) Close the dural incision with sutures.

(13) Provide an extradural drain tube always.

(14) Sew muscle, sew fascia, sew galea, sew skin.

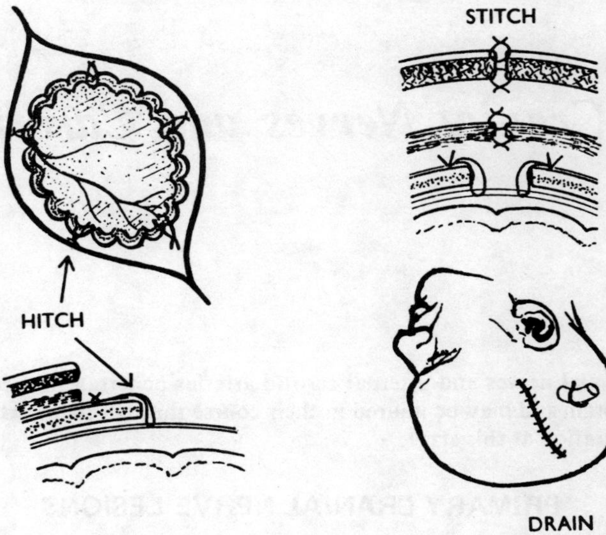

Problem Corner

You can't stop the bleeding?

(1) Hold something over it, and send for help.

(2) Pack it lightly and send the patient to help. Don't pack it firmly enough to reconstitute the pressure of the haematoma.

The dura remains depressed?

Lumbar puncture the patient and inject sterile saline until the dura approximates the skull. This unplugs the tentorial hernia and blows up the ventricles. (This is discussed more fully under chronic subdural haematoma.)

RECOMMENDED FURTHER READING

Hooper, R.S. (1954). 'Extradural Haemorrhages of the Posterior Fossa'. *Br. J. Surg.* **42,** 19

– (1959). 'Observations on Extradural Haemorrhage'. *Br. J. Surg.* **47,** 71

Jamieson, K.G. and Yelland, J.D.N. (1968). 'Extradural Haematoma'. *J. Neurosurg.* **29,** 13

McKissock, W., Taylor, J.C., Bloom, W.H. and Till, K. (1960). 'Extradural Haematoma'. *Lancet* **2,** 167

4—Cranial Nerves and Carotids

The cranial nerves and internal carotid arteries penetrate the coverings of the brain and may be injured in their course through them. Thus their consideration at this stage.

PRIMARY CRANIAL NERVE LESIONS

A lesion of a cranial nerve sustained at the moment of injury may be difficult to differentiate from nerve dysfunction occurring secondarily to intracranial haematomas.

Thus a primary nerve lesion may confuse the diagnostic picture, and the various nerve lesions now warrant comment.

Lest the number of nerves to be considered suggests an exhausting chapter, let us proceed by count-down, disposing of those least likely to be significant in head injury first.

Nerve Twelve

Because of its site, damage to the hypoglossal nerve rarely occurs in survivable injury.

Nerves Nine, Ten and Eleven

The glossopharyngeal, vagus and accessory nerves may rarely be injured by involvement in fractures traversing the jugular foramen, but injuries producing such lesions are again likely to be fatal.

Nerves Seven and Eight

These nerves, running a similar course from lateral pons through petrous temporal, are often involved together, though not necessarily so.

The mechanism is involvement by fracture, or shift of internal auditory meatus relative to brainstem.

The Facial Nerve

The nerve may be injured at the time of trauma and there results a lower neurone facial paresis. The outcome depends largely upon whether neurapraxia (recovery within days) axonotmesis (lesion in physical continuity), or neurotmesis (complete rupture) has occurred. Thus the nerve may recover completely within about ten days to three weeks, or show no sign of recovery for up to three months. Longer persistence of paralysis probably means neurotmesis, which is permanent.

In a second group, facial paralysis first appears at an interval after injury, due to oedema and swelling of the nerve within the fallopian canal. The onset is usually about three days after injury, and complete recovery is usual in about ten days.

Thus if the facial nerve lesion is delayed in onset, prognosis is good. If it is immediate, nothing should be done for the first three weeks, by which time some will have recovered, and it is too late to intervene in the rest. Intervention in any case is of doubtful value.

After three months, if no useful recovery has occurred, hypoglossal–facial anastomosis may be considered as a procedure giving a much superior functional result to fascial slings.

The Auditory Nerve

This nerve may be injured alone, or in conjunction with the facial, or the functions it subserves may be lost by damage to cochlea and vestibular apparatus.

Loss of hearing is usually permanent, but vestibular function may be substituted for by the other side. The more complex function of this nerve as compared with the facial makes the chances of recovery much less.

Nerves Three, Four and Six

These nerves, considered together because their courses are similar (from upper brainstem forward through cavernous sinus) may also be injured in a variety of ways:

(1) Involvement by fracture in a foramen of exit from the skull, the superior orbital fissure.

(2) Injury by shift of the petrous temporal, driven in by a crushing blow.

(3) Stretching when the skull, to which they are attached, moves suddenly in relation to their origin from brainstem.

(4) Avulsion from brainstem by the latter mechanism, commonly causing also brainstem injury.

Again, neurapraxia, axonotmesis or neurotmesis may occur. As a rough timetable, recovery is complete in ten days, incomplete in three months (though sometimes improving for years), or never occurs.

The Oculomotor Nerve

From the moment of injury there is a fixed dilated pupil. The pupilloconstrictor fibres are damaged and illumination of neither eye evokes response on the side of damage, while illumination of either eye evokes response on the normal side.

There are also external strabismus and paralysis of internal, upward and downward rotation, together with ptosis.

In the unconscious patient, fixed mydriasis and external strabismus are the usual findings.

Warning. The finding of unequal pupils may not mean either third nerve or optic nerve lesion. Other possibilities are:

(1) Traumatic mydriasis – eye injury.

(2) Brainstem dysfunction.

(3) Horner's syndrome; the abnormal pupil is the smaller. Note the pseudoptosis on the constricted side, the enophthalmos, the anhydrosis, and the cervical spine or brachial plexus traction injury which is responsible (the latter will cause paralysis of the arm contralateral to the larger pupil, and may easily deceive in the unconscious).

(4) Physiological inequality, or pre-existing disease.

(This section refers only to primary injury of the nerve. The most important cause of unequal pupils is compression of the oculomotor nerve secondary to intracranial haemorrhage, which will be discussed later.)

The Trochlear Nerve

Lesions of this nerve cannot be diagnosed in the unconscious, or not by the mere surgeon. They are often seen later in association with brainstem injury.

The Abducens Nerve

Internal strabismus or paralysis of abduction is present from the time of injury.

Nerve Five

The trigeminal nerve is rarely injured within the skull or in its passage through it. Damage to major divisions or branches of the nerve are more often seen in relation to injury of the facial bones.

Nerves One and Two

It must be remembered that the olfactory bulb and the optic nerve are portions of the brain not capable of repair in the sense that other nerves may be.

The Optic Nerve

The optic nerve may be injured within the optic canal by fracture through it, or by movement of brain within the skull and rupture of the nerve.

Blindness may be reported as a symptom or may be suspected from the pupillary reaction to light. Illumination of the affected eye evokes pupillary response in neither eye, while illumination of the other eye evokes pupillary response in both (contrast the findings with oculomotor nerve lesions!). The pupil of the blind eye may be large at first; don't confuse with the fixed dilated pupil of third nerve damage.

Blindness may not occur at the time of the injury, but may be delayed in some cases. Compare the optic nerve with the spinal cord in traumatic paraplegia. The possibilities are:

(1) Transection at the time of injury causes immediate and permanent blindness.

(2) Partial transection causes varieties of quadrantic loss (compare the Brown-Séquard syndrome).

(3) Neurapraxia can occur, causing temporary blindness like 'spinal shock'.

(4) Delayed blindness.

A fracture through the optic canal (which commonly accompanies a blow on the frontal eminence) may cause haemorrhage, and oedema of the nerve within it. This is the most important situation surgically, for immediate decompression of the nerve may save sight (progressive paralysis after spine injury is *the* indication for decompressive laminectomy, in the same way). In order to recognize the indication for decompression, one must know that sight has deteriorated at an interval. Look for the signs when the site of trauma and fracture suggest the possibility. The postion is urgent and this is a task for the expert.

Remember that lesions of optic tracts or radiations may also cause quadrantic loss, but this will be bilateral.

Papilloedema may cause consecutive optic atrophy, but papilloedema of this degree is rare in head injury.

The Olfactory Nerve

The most common lesion here is avulsion of the olfactory bulb from the brain – or from the cribriform plate – by cerebral shift. Such lesions are irreparable and result in anosmia together with loss of the olfactory modalities of what is commonly called 'taste'. All that may be left are the four modalities of taste *per se* – salt, sour, sweet and acid.

Injury to the small olfactory nerves traversing the cribriform plate may be recoverable, and may cause unpleasant parosmia which is continuous and not to be confused with the intermittent olfactory aura of temporal lobe epilepsy.

VESSELS

Carotico-cavernous Fistula

The particular vessel for consideration is the internal carotid. A fracture through the body of the sphenoid may tear this vessel as it lies in the cavernous sinus. There results a carotico-cavernous fistula.

The leading symptom of this is a bruit. If the patient complains of hearing noises, see if you can hear them before referring him to a psychiatrist. Listen over the orbits – use a bell stethoscope and have the patient open the other eye to stop the noise of blinking.

As the arteriovenous leak becomes established other symptoms and signs appear:

First a chemosis and then a proptosis–
The eye pulsates and eyesight abates,
For venous congestion may cause a suggestion
Of papilloedema, and then the fates
May decree that the other, the first eye's brother,
Shall also protrude (the picture's a rude
Bilat. exophthalmos, physicians can almost
Conclude that the thyroid is overimbued.)
The nose becomes stuffy, the eyelids are puffy
(Large veins can be felt in the lids),
Earache may be shocking (eustachian blocking),
The patient can't hear right for quids,
Then there's no improvement, the ocular movement
Is upset and he gets a squint,
For the nerve called abducent gets little amusement

From pressure in sinus – a hint
That third nerve may also be squashed in the wall so
The picture's ophthalmoplegia.
The hemisphere's starved, for blood flow is halved,
(With the shunt, there's none left to feed ya)
So gross mental slowing may also come owing
To increasing cer'bral ischaemia.
The limbs become weak, he may not now speak
And so becomes dreamier and dreamier,
Compress the carotid, if the lesion you've spotted,
The bruit will cease on the minute,
The eye will recede, ligation indeed
Is the treatment, if nothing's agin it.

Management

The diagnosis is usually confirmed by angiography and then the appropriate internal carotid artery is ligated in the neck. This is usually quite safe after about three weeks, when cross-circulation is well established.

If the bruit persists, due to intracranial cross-circulation from the other carotid, or anastomosis from the external carotid via the ophthalmic artery, the appropriate internal carotid artery is then ligated intracranially just below the ophthalmic. This latter manoeuvre is likely to improve the cerebral circulation by preventing loss of blood through the shunt.

RECOMMENDED FURTHER READING

Hamby, W. (1964). 'Carotid – Cavernous Fistula'. *J. Neurosurg.* **21**, 859
Hooper, R.S. (1951). 'Orbital Complications of Head Injury'. *Br. J. Surg.* **39**, 126

Part II
The Brain

When a blow falls on the scalp, how is its energy transmitted to the brain?

There are three primary mechanisms of injury.

Local Trauma

This we have already considered briefly under the subject of depressed fracture. The area of brain immediately beneath the site of impact may be injured by temporary or definitive skull deformity.

Local contusion or laceration of the brain may thus occur.

In the case of penetrating injury, much depends on the force of the blow. A high velocity bullet, for example, may cause widespread brain injury during its passage with almost explosive effect.

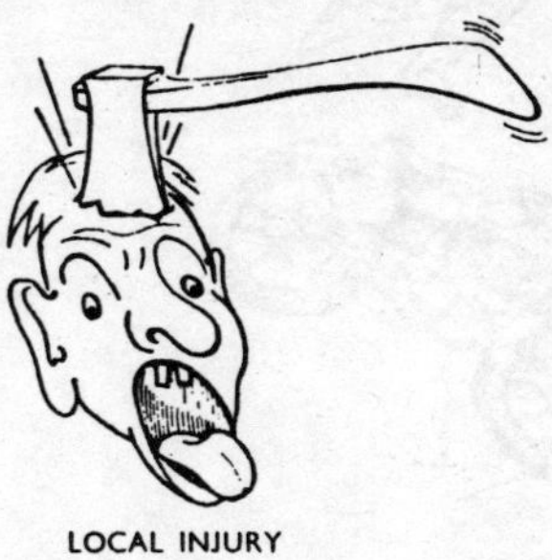

LOCAL INJURY

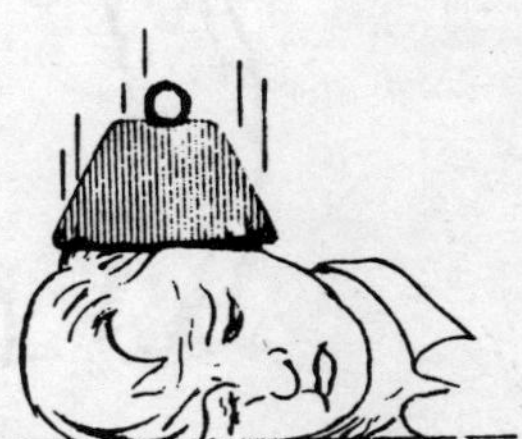

CRUSH

Crush Injury

Here the head remains stationary while compressed between two opposing forces; classically the railway truck buffers. The most important feature is the lack of movement. Gross skull fractures may occur and the petrous temporals may be driven inward, shearing as many as the third to eighth nerves inclusive, bilaterally. Yet consciousness is usually not lost and brain damage may not occur.

If the patient is unconscious as the result of a stationary crush injury, then deformity and brain damage have been extreme. Concussion does not occur in this type of injury.

Acceleration–Deceleration Injury

This is the usual traffic accident injury. The mechanism may also be associated with local trauma in falls or blows on the head from weapon or ball.

The significant feature is that the head is accelerated or decelerated.

It is in this group only that concussion occurs, and this mechanism is also responsible for the gross widespread brain damage which is a feature of the modern injury.

This mechanism we shall consider in more detail.

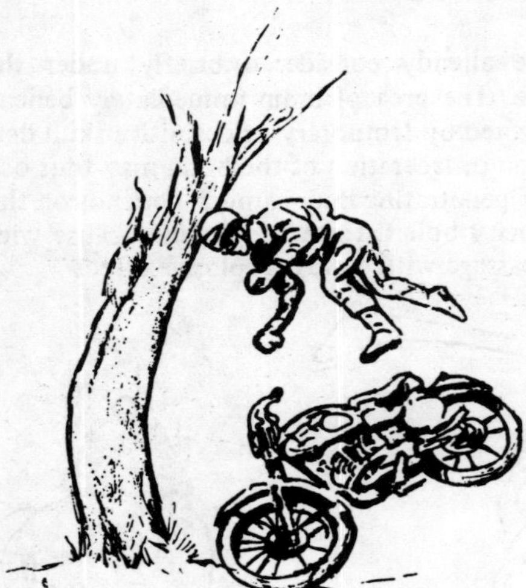

DECELERATION

5—*Injury to the Brain Surface*

Have you ever stamped on the brake pedal, cursing the incompetence of the other driver and remarking that there are a lot of fools on the road?

You would then have seen how your passengers were thrown forward within the car, travelling onward with their unbraked momentum. You might have considered the necessity for safety design in cars; collapsible steering wheel, absence of protruding knobs, padded upper edge of dashboard, seat belts, and so on. The object of these features is to lessen the impact, to soften the blow and reduce the rate of deceleration, and as such they are commendable.

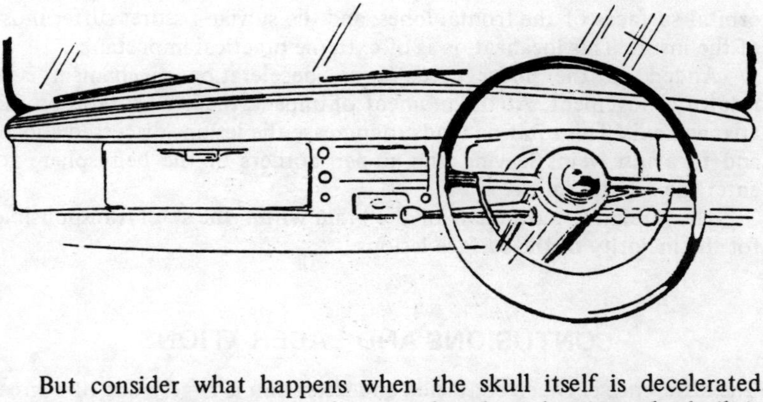

But consider what happens when the skull itself is decelerated. The soft brain then travels onward and crashes into the built-in dashboard that each of us owns, the knife-like sphenoidal ridges (complete with anterior clinoid projections), together with an unyielding facia of front wall of middle fossa, and a windscreen of rough orbital plates and frontal bone.

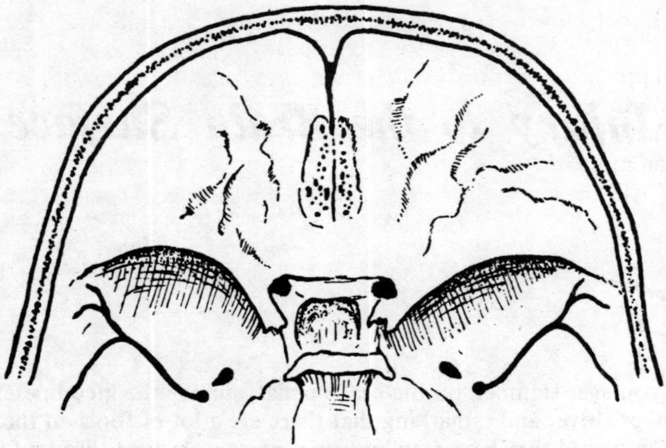

These are among the most lethal instruments known to Man, yet it is unlikely that their design can be modified, or their surfaces padded, in the foreseeable future!

When one looks inside a skull at these rough and sharp structures, one is not surprised that 90 per cent of cerebral lacerations and contusions occur in relation to them. The frontal and temporal poles, the orbital surfaces of the frontal lobes, and the sylvian fissures suffer most of the insult. This localization is of extreme practical importance.

Added to the linear acceleration–deceleration mechanism is a rotatory movement. At the moment of impact, the head rotates on the atlas and axis. This rotation tends to increase the lesions discussed above, and to avulse veins leaving the upper borders of the hemisphere to enter the sagittal sinus.

Thus, relative movement of the brain within the skull is responsible for the majority of the surface lesions.

CONTUSIONS AND LACERATIONS

The difference between contusion and laceration is largely one of degree. Clinical differentiation depends partly upon the degree of abnormality observed, and partly upon the presence of blood in the cerebrospinal fluid, as detected by the finding of neck stiffness or at lumbar puncture.

The immediate local neurological signs after injury are most commonly due to such contusions and lacerations. Once again, where are they?

INJURY TO THE BRAIN SURFACE

(1) Beneath the site of trauma, the 'coup' injury.

(2) Diametrically opposed to this, due to local change of intracranial pressure when the brain moves, the 'contrecoup' lesion.

(3) In the region of the sphenoidal ridge, the 'dashboard' injury.

(4) Along the superior border of the hemisphere, the rotatory vein – avulsion injury.

Of all these the sphenoidal ridge area is the most significant.

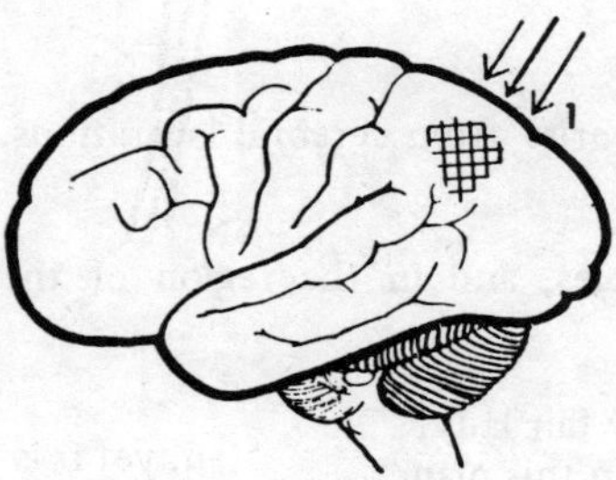

1 COUP

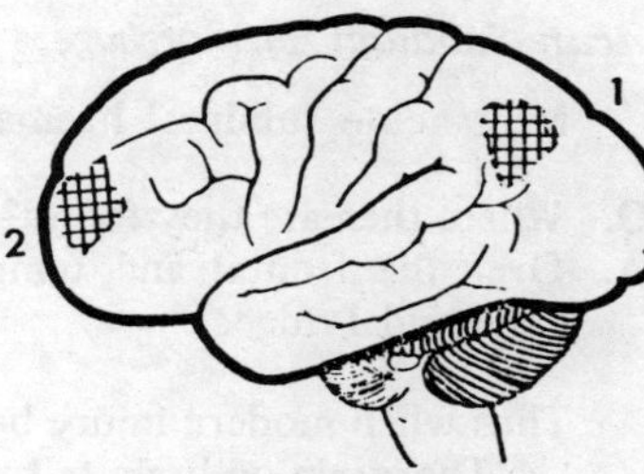

2 CONTRECOUP

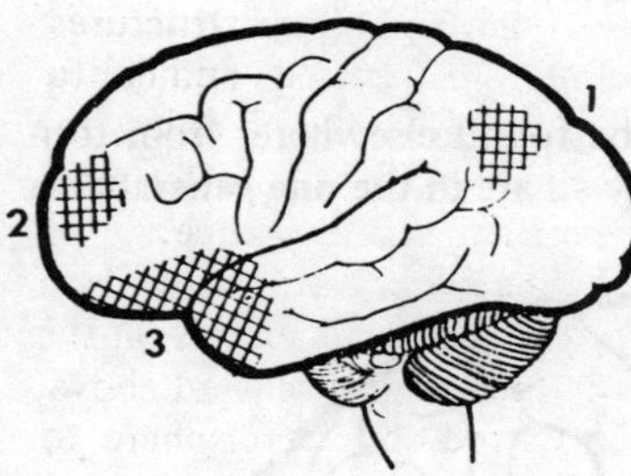

3 SPHENOIDAL RIDGE

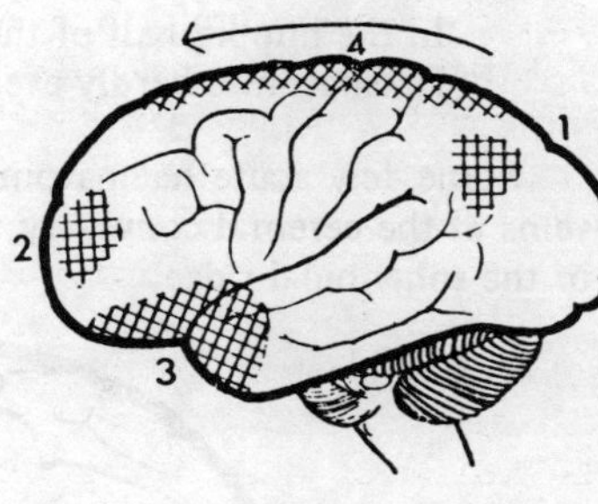

4 VEIN – AVULSION

HAEMORRHAGE AT THE BRAIN SURFACE

As the result of laceration, haemorrhage may occur, and at several levels.

Subarachnoid Haemorrhage

When a surface vessel is injured as it lies in the subarachnoid space, bleeding will probably occur. This may be immediate or delayed until initial contraction and retraction of vessels has subsided. The latter is a reactionary haemorrhage; 'delayed post-traumatic subarachnoid haemorrhage'. The effects are like those of spontaneous subarachnoid haemorrhage from a cerebral aneurysm, producing severe headache, stiff neck and photophobia, often with deterioration of consciousness. The volume of blood is insufficient of itself to raise the intracranial pressure significantly, but excessive secretion of cerebrospinal fluid from the perivascular spaces in response to the irritative blood may cause a secondary pressure rise.

Acute Subdural Haemorrhage

Most acute subdural haematomata arise from cerebral lacerations.

Q. Where then are they found?
A. Over the frontal and temporal poles, and in the region of the sphenoidal ridge.

Thus when modern injury befalls my fair lady,
'The strain on brain falls mainly in this plane'
while
'In the hupper half of the hemisphere,
Haematomas hardly ever happen'.

Some few acute haematomata may be found elsewhere, from torn veins at the cerebral convexity, but nearly all are in the one general area of the sphenoidal ridge.

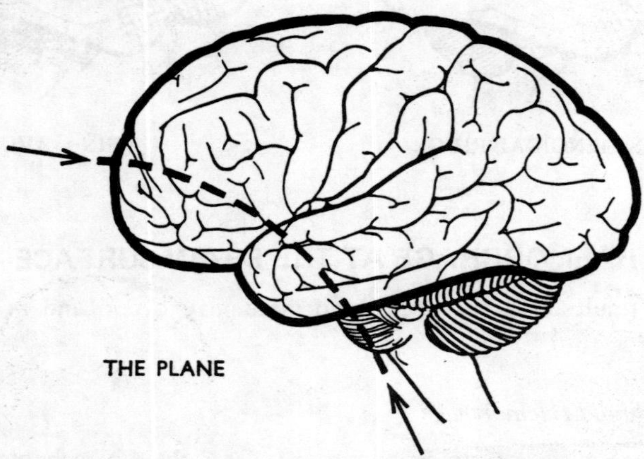

THE PLANE

It is as simple as that! (Chronic subdural haematoma, an entirely different condition, is considered later.)

Surface Intracerebral Haematoma

The surface laceration also determines the occurrence of surface intracerebral haematomata – the formation of a clot within the laceration, spreading into the brain on the one hand, and out into the subdural space on the other.

Q. Where are these to be found?
A. Nearly always in the orbital surface or pole of the frontal lobe, and in the temporal pole.

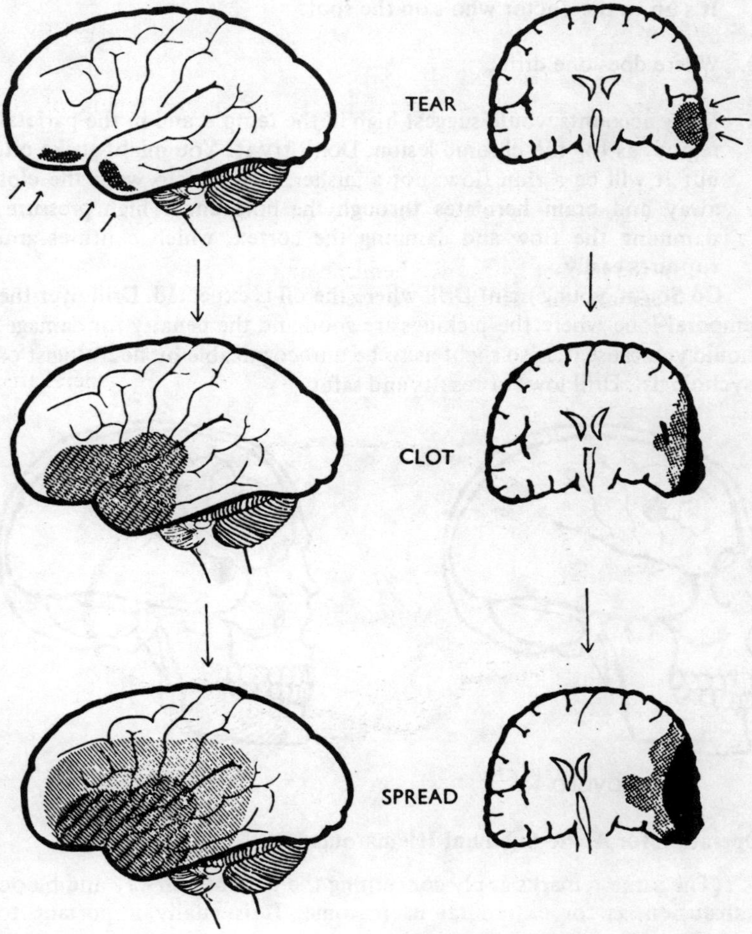

DRILLING THE HOLE

Let us defer again until later a description of the clinical course of these lesions and the means of diagnosis, and now consider the operation that is to be performed.

Q. Who drills the hole?
A. When injury's urban it's not so disturbin',
The neurosurgeon can let out the clot:
Acute subdural may often be rural –
It's up to the doctor who's on the spot.

Q. Where does one drill?

A. Many accounts would suggest high in the temple, and in the parietal region, as for the chronic lesion. Don't try it! You might strike oil, but it will be a thin flow, not a gusher. Attempt to wash the clot away and brain herniates through the hole under high pressure, damming the flow and damning the cortex, which contuses and ruptures easily.

Go South, young man! Drill where the oil is expected. Drill over the temporal lobe where the pickings are good and the penalty for damage, should you cause it, is so slight as to be unrecognizable by neurologist or psychologist. Drill low for results and safety.

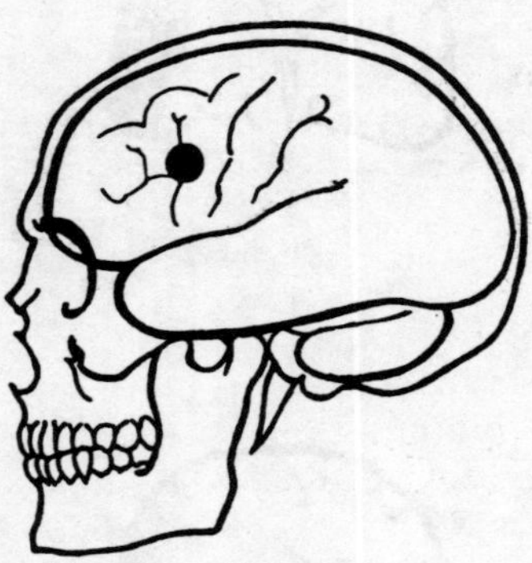

ILL ADVISED

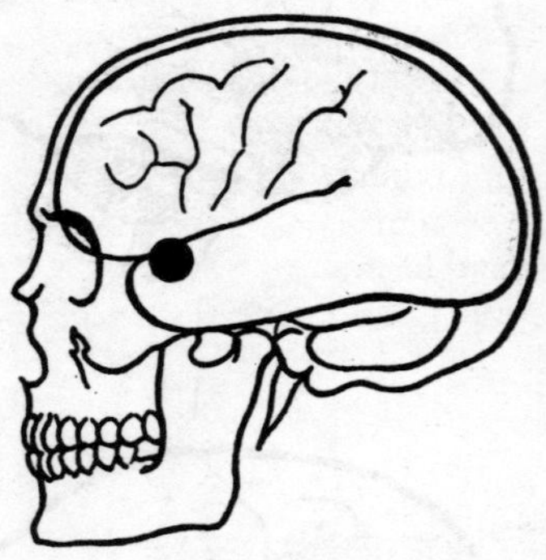

CORRECT

Operation for Acute Subdural Haematoma

(The same remarks apply concerning the patient's airway and blood transfusion as for extradural haematoma. It is vitally important to prepare your patient for operation, but not to waste time while you do this.)

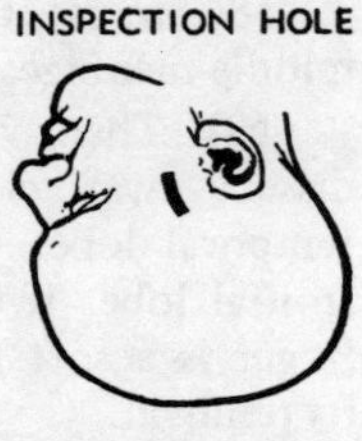

(1) Take roughly the midpoint between orbit and ear, just behind the hairline, and plan a hole just comfortable above the zygomatic arch. Mark the incision vertically before you drape.

(2) Drill an inspection hole, 2·5 cm incision, straight to bone, temporalis scraped back, retractor haemostasis, as for the extradural.

(3) Open the dura and see what you find. If no blood, there may be a collection of cerebrospinal fluid under pressure. This means arachnoid tear, and the haematoma may not be far away. If no collection, what is the pressure? If high, the haematoma must be elsewhere – beyond the hole (depress the cortex and seek blood; if you find it, pursue it), or on the other side (close the hole).

(4) If you find blood, wash away a little, depress the cortex with a dissector or a thin spatula, and see whence it comes. From below over the temporal lobe? From above and in front over the frontal lobe?

(5) Enlarge the incision appropriately; up and down for temporal lobe, or curving forward for frontal lobe. (For the latter, cut directly from temporal crest to above the eye to form a triangular flap, or curve the incision behind the hairline for cosmetic nicety.)

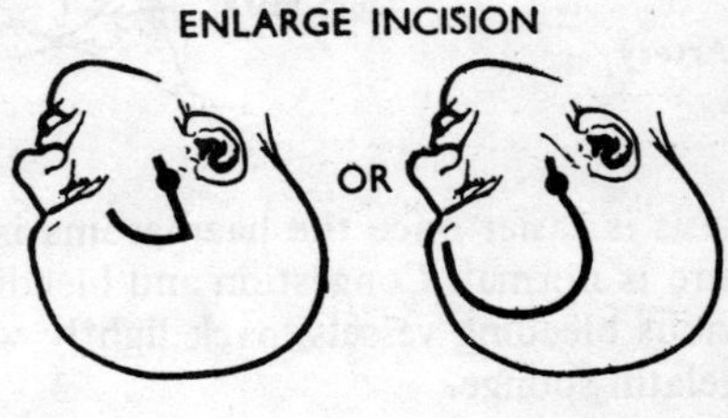

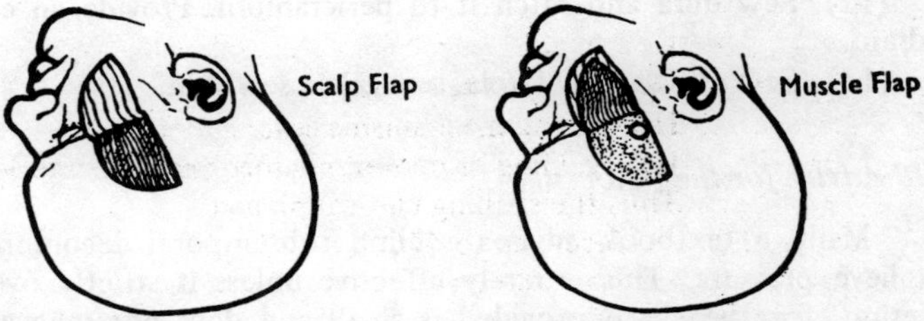

(6) Scrape the whole front half of the temporalis from the bone and drape it over zygoma.

(7) Remove all the bone of the anterior temporal fossa, right up to the temporal crest. Take the outer end of the sphenoidal ridge.

(8) Incise the dura to expose the clot, in cruciate fashion. The middle meningeal artery will have to be secured.

(9) Then wash away, suck away and dissect away clot, until you can see the temporal lobe, the sylvian fissure and the frontal lobe. If clot is tenacious, the gloved finger is a soft and sensitive instrument for its removal.

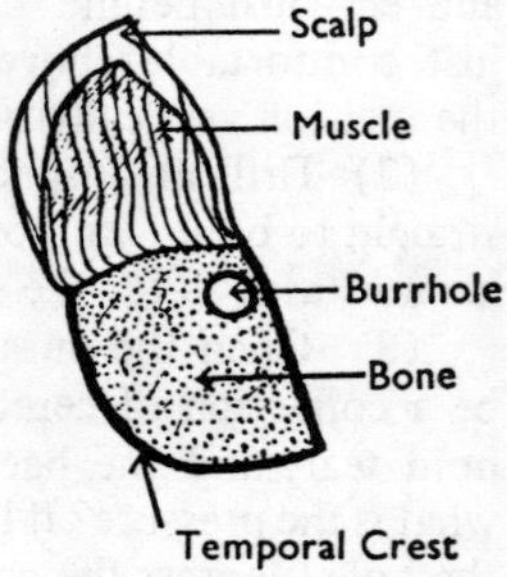

(10) Seek the bleeding point, and thus the cortical tear. Clot may lie within it, or pulped brain may exude from it. Gently suck these away.

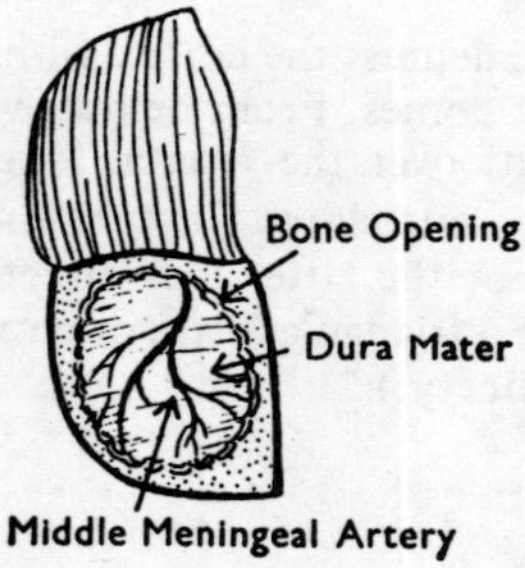

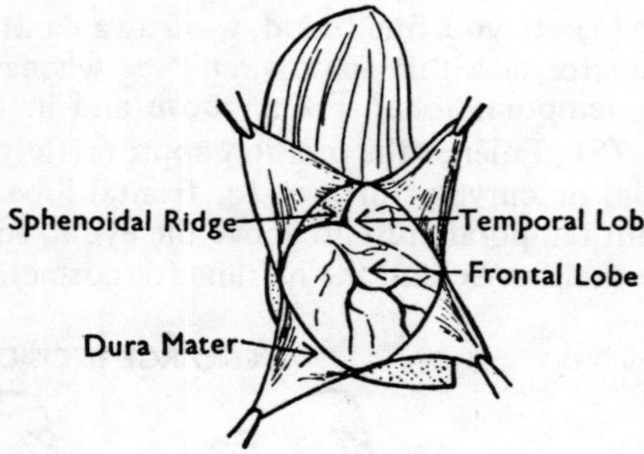

(11) Haemostasis is easier once the haematoma is removed and the intracranial pressure is normal. Congestion and bleeding subside. Ligate or diathermy obvious bleeding vessels, pack lightly with wet wool and wait. Dress with gelatin sponge.

(12) Sew dura and hitch it to pericranium. Provide an extradural drain.

(13) Sew muscle, sew fascia, sew galea, sew skin.

Ill Advice for the Innocent

Many a textbook advises a blind subtemporal decompression to relieve pressure. This is rarely effective unless it strictly overlies the lesion, for the space provided is small and does not relieve cerebral distortion unless it chances to be correctly sited. The advice is pertinent only to those who don't know where to look for the lesion!

RECOMMENDED FURTHER READING

McKissock, W., Richardson, A. and Bloom, W.H. (1960). 'Subdural Haematoma'. *Lancet* **1**, 1365

6—Injury to the Brain in Depth

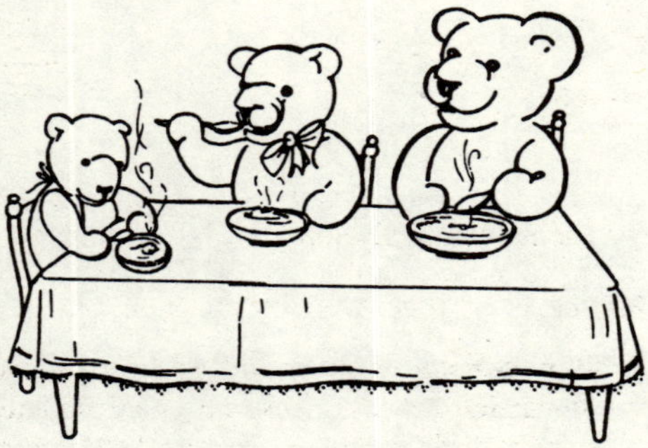

In winter my children eat porridge.
This is a habit which I find distasteful, not necessarily because it reminds me of the atheroma which might be engendered by the blob of cream in the middle.

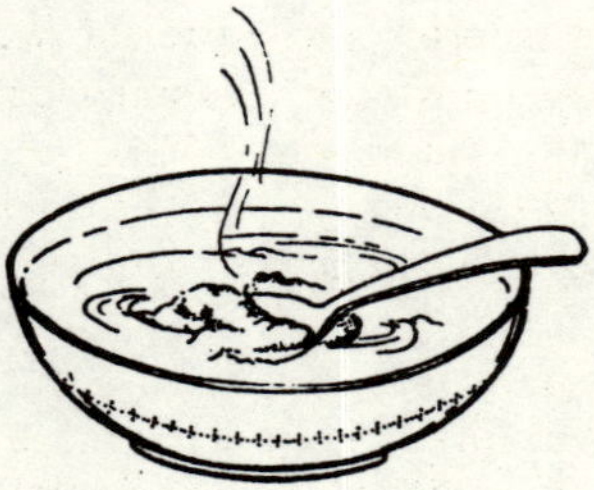

But if I strike the edge of a plate, I see the porridge slop about slightly, while a ripple disturbs its surface. If I spin the plate, the blob of of cream lags behind, and only gradually catches up with the rest. Thus shearing stresses are created between succesive layers of porridge.

The consistency of the brain is not dissimilar, and these are the mechanisms of injury to the brain in depth, when the skull is suddenly shifted. Linear or rotatory acceleration–deceleration injury sets up shearing stresses throughout the brain. Fibre tract slides on fibre tract, capsule on radiation. Axons may be disrupted, and small vessels crossing shear lines may be torn, giving rise to widespread petechial haemorrhages.

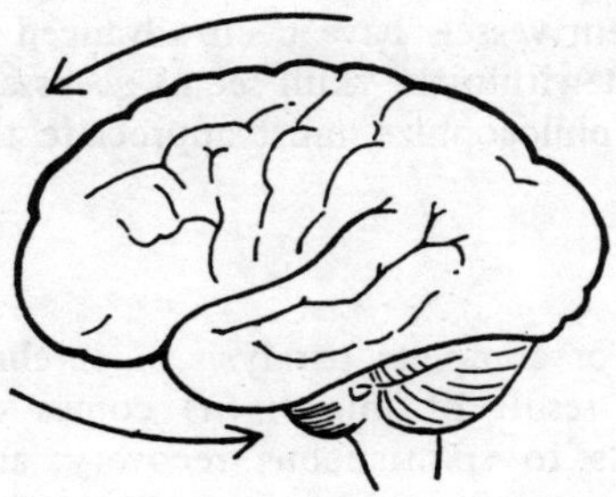

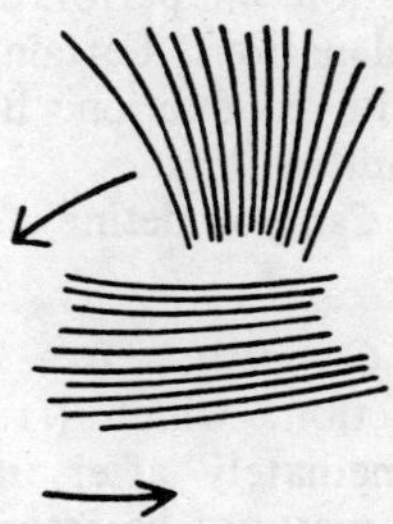

So much for the mechanical factor.

The Vascular Factor

When the brain moves suddenly it does so upon a leash consisting of cerebral vessels and cranial nerves. These may be long and redundant, or so short as to be a veritable tether. In the latter case they may be suddenly stretched and even avulsed from the brain (these built-in seat belts that might protect the brain from the sphenoidal dashboard injury in fact increase the danger).

The vessels most liable to injury in this fashion are the smallest; paradoxically the most important also. The basal perforating arteries, passing through the anterior and posterior perforated substances from the anterior, middle and posterior cerebral arteries, and vessels supplying the brainstem, are quite vulnerable.

Traction upon these vessels may cause spasm, as the non-gentle neurosurgeon knows to his patient's cost, resulting in ischaemia of their territory of supply.

Thus arise multiple widespread lesions of the brain in depth, due to mechanical and vascular factors. It is important that one has a clear and graphic picture of this state if one is to treat it correctly. In the next chapter we shall consider the effects of injury to special vital areas of brain.

Concussion

Concussion occurs only in the acceleration–deceleration injury. To this extent it may be said to be an acceleration phenomenon. In the experimental animal a threshold level of acceleration, below which concussion cannot occur, may be demonstrated.

There are many theories as to the cause of concussion, the mechanism of which is still not known. 'Commotio cerebri', sudden cerebrospinal fluid shock wave down the aqueduct, brainstem traction, and traction on perforating and brainstem vessels have been advanced as explanations. Certainly cerebral shift within the skull seems necessary to its production. But many who philosophize most appreciate the condition least.

Can you define it?

Concussion is a state of partial or complete paralysis of cerebral function, which (*i*) occurs as the result of injury; (*ii*) comes on immediately after injury; (*iii*) tends to spontaneous recovery; and (*iv*) may not be associated with any macroscopic or microscopic lesion of brain.

Note especially: tends immediately after injury to spontaneous recovery.

Thus there is no such thing as delayed concussion, and no such thing as progressive deterioration due to concussion.

Note also that the severity of injury is best assessed by the presence or absence of concussion, and its duration and effects. The most readily estimated features of concussion in the clinical history are:

(1) The presence and duration of unconsciousness (though other factors enter here).

(2) The presence and duration of retrograde amnesia.

If the patient remembers all details of the accident (and is not just reciting a hearsay account), he has no retrograde amnesia and was *not* significantly concussed.

If the patient did not lose consciousness he was *not* concussed (speak of subconcussive states if you must, but don't confuse concussion).

Consciousness

Q. What is consciousness?

A. The answer varies from philosopher to poet, from clinician to electrophysiologist.

Q. What clinically is consciousness?

A. It is a state of accessibility of the patient to question or command verbal or otherwise.

Q. Where is consciousness determined in the brain?

A. The obvious answer seemed to be 'in the cerebral cortex', for this is the 'highest' layer of brain; but it has only recently been acquired, as a refinement, and consciousness is much more basic. Certainly cortex is necessary for most of those functions by which we recognise consciousness clinically, but large areas of cortex can be removed without disturbing consciousness.

Q. Is consciousness then dependent upon a certain quorum of cerebral activity, present at the meeting?

A. No, for isolated lesions in hypothalamus and upper brainstem may cause unconsciousness without injury to the rest of the brain.

Q. Do these lesions merely de-afferent the cortex by dividing fibre tracts? Do they thus reduce activity below a quorum?

A. No, they affect a particular structure, the brainstem reticular formation.

Q. What is the function of this reticular formation?

A. It is the alerting mechanism of the brain, probably responsible for the scanning alpha rhythm of the electro-encephalogram, the presence of which is the electrophysiologist's definition of consciousness.

When consciousness is lost, the brainstem or hypothalamus is affected!

Q. Where is consciousness determined in the brain?

A. You have your answer.

RECOMMENDED FURTHER READING

Denny-Brown, D. and Russell, W.R. (1941). 'Experimental Cerebral Concussion'. *Brain* **64**, 93

Holbourn, A.H.S. (1943). 'Mechanics of Head Injuries'. *Lancet* **2**, 438

Ommaya, A.K. (1966). 'Trauma to the Nervous System'. *Ann. R. Coll. Surg.* **39**, 317

Wright, R.D. (1944). 'Concussion and Contusion'. *Surgery, St. Louis* **15**, 661

– (1946). 'Concussion and Contusion'. *Surgery, St. Louis* **19**, 661

7—Special Brain Sites

'One of the major recent advances in our concept of head injury has been the categorisation of certain syndromes specific to injury of particular cerebral structures . . . . '

That seems a deadly enough opening to a discussion of vital functions! But please read on and we will keep it light.

Four highly rated suburbs of the cerebral metropolis require reassessment:

- the hypothalamus
- the brainstem
- the frontal lobe
- the temporal bone

THE HYPOTHALAMUS

Primary stress injury here may cause special disturbances of vital function: (*i*) neurogenic hyperthermia; (*ii*) gastric erosion; (*iii*) diabetes insipidus; and (*iv*) somnolent obesity.

Neurogenic Hyperthermia

Excessive fever due to hypothalamic disorder is of great importance in the acute stage of injury. The patient may die in hyperpyrexia unless the state is recognized and treated early enough. The patient is usually unconscious, but not always.

Heat losing mechanisms cease function.

Heat gaining or conserving mechanisms function to excess.

Thus the striking clinical picture:

- fever, up to 42C°
- no sweating
- pilo-erection
- peripheral vasoconstriction
- tachypnoea
- circulatory collapse

In the fully developed state the picture is unmistakable. The patient has a hot dry trunk (no sweating), but cold dry face and limbs (no peripheral vasodilatation). There are 'goose-pimples' due to pilo-erection in an effort to conserve heat. Shivering may occur to produce heat.

The peripheral vasoconstriction may be so marked that the axillary temperature is 1°C below the oral, which in turn may be as much as 2°C below rectal or oesophageal temperature.

Thus *rectal* temperature must be measured for the recognition of this state.

In the early stages the respiratory rate is often increased, and this may be the earliest sign of impending trouble. Rapid respiration after head injury is always a reason for measuring rectal temperature. Respiration becomes increasingly rapid until the early hyperventilation gives way to rapid shallow breathing (up to 80 per minute) which produces almost no pulmonary ventilation. Dead space air only is exchanged.

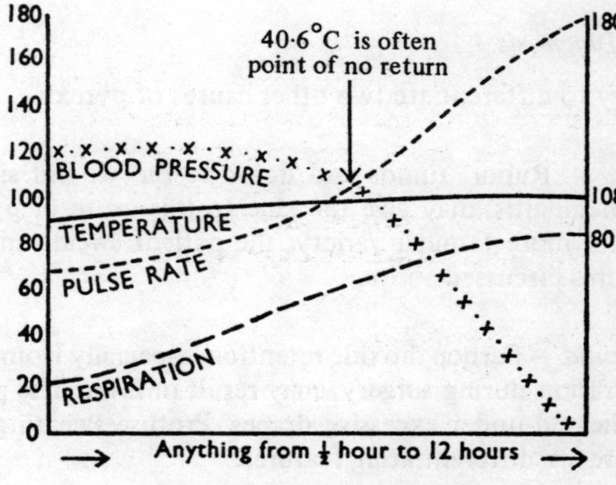

THE HYPERTHERMIC CRISIS

At first the circulation remains stable, but the pulse rate may rise. Later circulatory failure develops with rapid thin pulse, falling blood pressure and venous blotching on non-dependent areas of the limbs.

The whole process is a vicious circle. The higher the fever, the more rapid and inefficient the respiration becomes, and terminal circulatory failure approaches. The more frenzied and disordered the respiration, the higher the temperature goes.

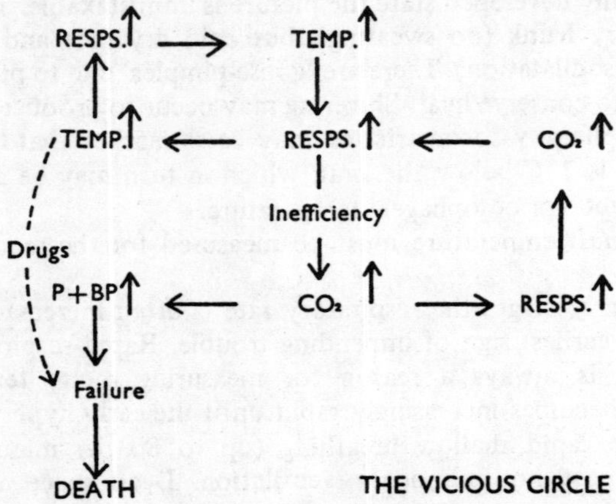

Rectal temperature measurement is essential for early diagnosis, and rapid respiration may be the first clue.

Differential Diagnosis

It is necessary to differentiate two other causes of pyrexia.

Infection. – Rubor, tumor and dolor at the wound site, or neck stiffness in meningitis, may give the clue to this cause of pyrexia. The fever is of the more familiar variety; the patient sweats and lacks the specific features discussed above.

Hypercapnia. – Carbon dioxide retention, especially from inadequate care of respiration during surgery, may result in fever. The patient may also be overheated under excessive drapes. Profuse sweating and raised blood pressure are differentiating features.

Treatment of Neurogenic Hyperthermia

Cool the patient.
37·5°C – remove blankets, heavy clothing and hot water bottles (which should not be used anyway.)
38·5°C – expose naked patient to draught of a fan.
39°C – sponge with iced water or spirit.
39·5°C – pack in ice bags – crushed ice in ordinary polythene bags. Apply them especially over major vessels in axillae and groins, and over the abdomen. Use plenty.

If the temperature can be kept below 40°C, the patient will probably survive, especially if his respiratory rate falls. If the temperature remains above 40°C from this cause, he will surely die.

More heroic endeavours sometimes needed include ice-cold gastric, rectal and intravenous fluid, but control should be possible before these are necessary.

Drugs

Aspirin may be administered liberally, and has proved helpful.

The homeopathic doses of morphia recommended by some (i.e., grains 1/32), constitute wishful thinking.

Largactil 50 mg to stop shivering is a most useful drug if shivering prevents cooling, but *don't* use except in small doses if peripheral failure is present or imminent. A rapid pulse rate, a falling blood pressure, increasing cyanosis, or poor capillary return in the limbs suggest this possibility. Even 25 mg may cause circulatory collapse at this stage.

Pethedine and Phenergan are to be rigorously eschewed for the same reason.

(A digression. The reverse state of hypothermia sometimes occurs, the hibernation syndrome. Do not accept an 'unrecordably' low temperature in neurosurgery. Use an ordinary thermometer instead of a clinical one. The temperature may be as low as 26·4°C, usually with unconsciousness, slow pulse, slow respiration, and low blood pressure. Warm this patient).

Gastric Erosion

Acute gastric erosion with haematemesis or melaena may result from hypothalamic dysfunction, even in the absence of aspirin as recommended above. Treat conservatively.

Diabetes Insipidus

Injury to the 'hypothalamic-hypophyseal axis' may cause diabetes insipidus. Usually there is a major fracture of the skull base.

Polyuria does not appear for two or three days, often persists for two or three months, and tends to recover spontaneously.

Beware dehydration in the unconscious.

Pitressin tannate in oil or pituitary snuff may be given.

Somnolent Obesity

This, the 'hypothalamic syndrome', is an occasional end result of injury. Consult the endocrinologists about this!

THE BRAINSTEM

The brainstem may be injured by:

Stretching of peduncles when hemispheres shift.

Deceleration against basisphenoid and dorsum sellae.

Lateral shift of peduncle against tentorial margin.

Stretch or avulsion from it of cranial nerves.

Traction on its vascular supply.

Various clinical pictures may develop, according to the level of injury.

Unconsciousness

This is as common as one would expect from injury to the brainstem reticular formation. It may be very prolonged, and require special endeavours to awaken and alert the patient.

Treatment of Prolonged Unconsciousness

Once the patient's state has become stable, measures to awaken him may include:

Drugs. Benzedrine in dosage of 10 mg a.m., and 5 mg noon, increasing to up to 30 and 20 or more if tolerated, may help to restore a normal diurnal waking and nocturnal sleeping rhythm.

Activity. The patient should be stimulated often, by feeding him by mouth even if this is slow, by sitting him out of bed, and by physiotherapy.

Neurogenic Hyperthermia

This may occur from midbrain and high pontine lesions, and is the same condition as discussed above.

Ocular Signs

Lesions of midbrain by avulsion of cranial nerves (notably the third) may display evidence of injury both of the cranial nerve involved and of the quadrigeminal plate.

Supranuclear palsy results in defective co-ordination of the eyes. Conjugate movement may be lost (especially the upward) and rotatory nystagmus may develop. Irregularities of pupillary size are common, and may fluctuate rapidly. Pinpoint pupils occur with pontine lesions.

Since the third nerve traverses the red nucleus, the coarse intention tremor due to injury of the latter may occur in association with oculomotor lesions. This tends to resolve only after the lapse of months or years.

Decerebrate Rigidity

This state may occur from lesions anywhere between the red nucleus in the midbrain and the lateral vestibular nucleus in mid-pons The lesion may be anatomical, such as caused by haemorrhage, or a physiological and recoverable transection.

Features are rigid extension of the trunk and lower limbs, which internally rotate and, with physiologically extended and adducted feet, assume the posture of cerebral diplegia. Opisthotonos may occur. The arms are held rigidly extended and internally rotated by the sides with adducted and flexed wrist and fingers, or rigidly flexed across the chest. This state represents tonic spasm of all antigravity muscles, including the masseters.

This decerebrate rigidity may occur in spasms associated with circulatory and respiratory disturbance.

Righting Reflexes

Righting reflexes are occasionally seen in association with decerebrate rigidity. They are chiefly of academic interest since those exhibiting them rarely survive. The most common are those evoked by neck rotation, the jaw limbs extending and the occipital limbs flexing. Sometimes stepping reflexes may be elicited.

Flaccidity

When the lesion is below the vestibular nucleus (in lower pons and medulla) or when the whole brainstem is involved as in concussion, complete flaccidity is the common picture.

Circulation and Respiration

Injury to the lower brainstem may cause disturbance of the circulatory and respiratory centres, resulting in cardiac and respiratory dysrhythmias and hypotension. Of these, more later; and note that they may occur in spasms related to those of decerebrate rigidity.

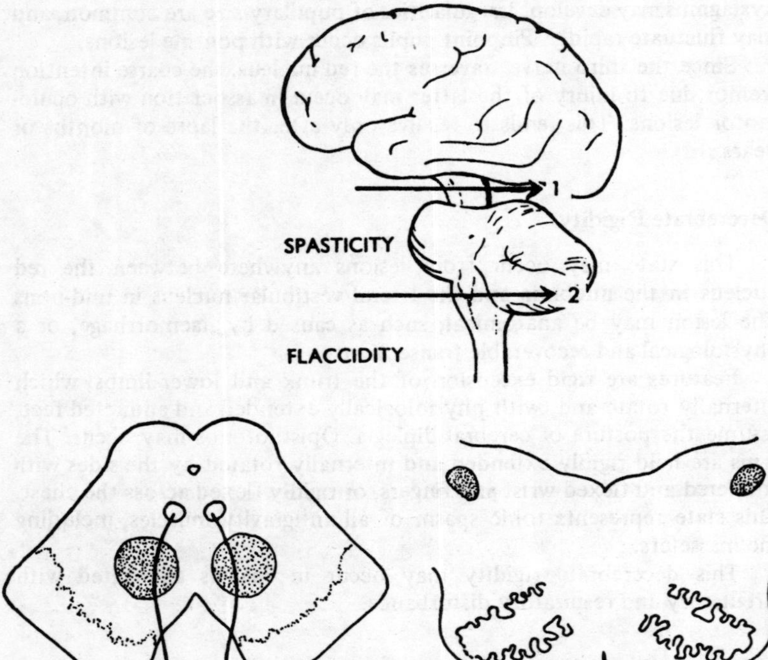

1 RED NUCLEUS AND 3RD NERVE 2 LATERAL VESTIBULAR NUCLEI

Treatment

Cool the patient who suffers decerebrate spasms. The spasms are due to a rapidly changing state in the brainstem. Small vessels may be injured and constricted, and oedema and contusions contribute to tissue anoxia. Little can be done to increase the oxygen supply to damaged brain through damaged vessels, but the oxygen requirement of brain can be reduced to the level of the supply available.

For every 1°C of fever that the patient develops (and fever is common with brainstem injury) his basal metabolism (and oxygen requirement) rises 10 per cent. At 30°C, his oxygen requirement will fall to only half the normal.

By cooling him from 39° to 30°C, you reduce his oxygen need well over 50 per cent.

Pack him in plastic bags of crushed ice; give Largactil if necessary to stop shivering (with caution if blood pressure is low). Prevention of shivering is important since shivering not only raises the temperature but also causes gross increase of oxygen consumption by as much as 200 per cent.

Steadying of respiration and cessation of spasms indicate success.

THE FRONTAL LOBES

It has been seen that the frontal lobes are often injured in the 'sphenoidal dashboard' injury. Two important aspects are:

Personality effects.

Electrolyte effects.

Personality Effects

Damage to the frontal lobes may simulate the effect of leucotomy, conservative or radical. In the early stages the effect may vary from mild loss of inhibition, to ribaldry when wit is retained, to vulgar obscenity.

One must be constantly wary of resenting and even neglecting a patient whose obscenity of speech and behaviour is the consequence of his injury. One must also resist the tendency to give excessive sedatives to these patients to their detriment for the sake of peace.

The situation should be understood by those called upon to nurse the patient. In a few weeks or months, when reserve has been regained, they may not recognize and might even admire their previously despised charge.

Electrolyte Effects

The orbital and medial surfaces of the frontal lobes constitute the highest (cortical) level of the autonomic nervous system. Injury here, or to the anterior cerebral arteries which supply the area, may result in bizarre changes.

Cerebral 'salt hoarding' is the commonest state, producing hypernatraemia and hyperchloraemia, often with a raised blood urea level. In others hyperkalaemia may occur.

It is not certain whether these are primary cerebral effects. Other arguments concern dietary change, dehydration, and respiratory alkalosis. But in some cases peculiar deterioration of the patient will be accounted for by odd electrolyte imbalance.

THE TEMPORAL LOBES

The temporal lobes may also be injured by the 'sphenoidal dashboard' mechanism, or their uncinate processes may be damaged, together with the brainstem, against the tentorial edges. Two important aspects of such injuries are memory disturbance, and effects on the rhinencephalon.

Memory Disturbance

Bilateral temporal lobe damage commonly causes severe disturbance of memory, either transiently or permanently.

When concussion occurs the last afferent stimuli experienced do not achieve recording in memory, by whatever mechanism that may occur, before consciousness is lost. Thus retrograde amnesia is a feature of concussion and its duration is a measure of the severity of injury. When consciousness returns memory may not function normally for some time, so that post-traumatic amnesia occurs and its duration is also a measure of the severity of injury.

In severe injury, long term disorder of memory is common. Long-past events may be remembered clearly, but memory for recent events may not be established. Such a disability may disqualify patients from any employment for they are incapable of consecutive activity in even the simplest routines. This handicap, together with effects of frontal lobe damage on personality which may prohibit normal social intercourse (even harmonious existence in the family circle), constitutes one of the gravest and least manageable of all disabilities that may afflict patients otherwise in sound physical health.

The Rhinencephalon

Many patients suffering brainstem injury exhibit involuntary chewing movements not related to olfactory or gustatory stimuli. These probably represent abnormal motor output from the damaged uncinate processes.

RECOMMENDED FURTHER READING

Hooper, R.S. (1964). *Neurosurgical Nursing,* (pp. 126, 127). Springfield, Ill.: Thomas

Strich, S.J. (1956). 'Diffuse Degeneration of the Cerebral White Matter in Severe Dementia Following Head Injury.' *J. Neurol. Neurosurg. Psychiat.* **19**, 163

8—The Primary Neurological State

After examining the patient's head one should set about assessing the neurological state due to the primary injuries. This represents the baseline from which improvement, or deterioration due to the occurrence of a complication, can be gauged.

This primary neurological state of the patient should be assessed in the light of what is already known of the type and site of injury, and its likely effects on brain and nerves.

Two over-riding factors are of importance: concussion and surgical shock.

Concussion

This temporary paralytic state may mask the less transitory signs of definitive damage. Only as concussion recedes may localizing signs become evident. Thus if localizing signs first appear when the patient is improving, do not regard them necessarily as signs of deterioration.

Surgical Shock

This is uncommon in head injury unless there has been excessive blood loss from scalp, or other injury to trunk or limb, but in its presence neurological examination may be invalid.

STATE OF CONSCIOUSNESS

The first requirement is accurate assessment of the state of consciousness of the patient. The terminology used must be such as to permit of accuracy. The commonly adopted convention in terminology is:

ALERTNESS: Fully orientated and mentally agile.

CONFUSION: Awake and capable of conversation, but disorientated in time or place.

STUPOR: Drowsy, but can be roused with difficulty to converse at simple level.

SEMICOMA: Inaccessible to verbal or other question or command, but responding to pain.

COMA: Not responding to painful stimuli except perhaps by change of respiratory rhythm.

However, usage of these terms is so variable from doctor to doctor and nurse to nurse, that they are better avoided. You may know what you mean, but will others? The range of semicoma is extensive; cannot one be more accurate?

Note exactly your observation, and insist on the nursing staff doing the same. For example:

'Alert, orientated'.

'Knows who he is, not time or place'.

'Knows where he is, not day or time'.

'Inaccurate answers to simple questions, e.g., . . .'

'Answers yes or no only'.

'Swears only'.

'Obeys commands, but won't answer'.

'Won't obey commands, slaps may hand if I pinch him'.

'Pulls hand away if I pinch it'.

'Slides hand away sluggishly if I pinch it'.

'Brisk shrug response to pain'.

'Sluggish extensor response to pain'.

'Barely perceptible response to pain'.

'No response to painful stimuli'.

If such recordings were faithfully kept, we should all know where we are. Deterioration or improvement would be easy to assess.

Note

The best response that can be elicited, by fair means or foul, is to be recorded.

'Sleeping' should never be recorded – the chief difference between sleep and coma is that the sleeper can be awakened.

'Responds to painful stimuli' is a grossly inadequate report – the fully conscious patient does, as does the almost dead.

'Restlessness, irritability', and so on, should not be recorded as states of consciousness, but noted as additional phenomena. Full consciousness may be associated with extreme irritability in some individuals as a normal state.

ASSESSMENT OF THE UNCONSCIOUS PATIENT

Please put down that tendon hammer. You will achieve much more by looking, and with your empty hands!

Cranial Nerves

One: can't be assessed.

Two: if appropriate light reflexes are absent on stimulation of one eye, present on stimulation of the other, there may be an optic nerve lesion.

Even if the patient can't answer, test visual fields grossly by: (*i*) light reflex with torch shone from either side; (*ii*) blink in response to menace (threatened blow with a fist from either side – but don't cause a wind on cornea and corneal reflex). Gross hemianopia may thus be picked. Examine the fundi.

Three: pupil size and light reflexes.

Three, four and six: are eyes conjugate? If not, is strabismus due to one particular nerve? Is there conjugate deviation? (Stimulated frontal lobe eye fields cause conjugate deviation to opposite side, paralysed frontal eyefield to same side). Are eyes roving? If not, rock head from side to side. Eyes may fix on an external object, and then movements can be assessed as head moves.

Five: painful stimuli to face – any response?

Seven: observe facial tone carefully. Press on each supra-orbital nerve in turn and watch reflex movement on face.

Eight: cannot assess in the unconscious.

Nine to twelve: rarely injured, hard to assess. Don't trouble.

General

Posture

Is there the extensor rigidity of brainstem injury?
Is there flaccidity?
Is there opisthotonos?
Is there neck stiffness?

Tone

Compare upper limb with upper limb, lower with lower. Flex and straighten limb, lift and drop it. If different, which is abnormal? Note especially flaccidity of paralysis or of cerebellar damage, and spasticity of paralysis in other cases. Gross spasticity suggests brainstem injury which may be unilateral. Is there clonus?

Movement

Look for spontaneous movement. Is it noticeably absent in any one limb, or on one side?

Stimulate reflex movement of each limb; pinch them and watch quality of movement. Is there a localizing deficiency?

Reflexes

Use your car key for the plantars, elicit the Hoffman's.

Then take up the tendon hammer if you wish to add the minor frills to the information you have.

ASSESSMENT OF THE CONSCIOUS

Again save that tendon hammer for the end. Ask about:

Headache.
Vision.
Hearing.

Examine fully neurologically. Special points are:

(1) The visual fields.

Don't neglect these for they may give information regarding the optic nerves, chiasm, tracts, radiations through temporal and parietal lobes, and the occipital visual cortex. This is a long axis of brain that cannot be examined with a tendon hammer!

(2) Conjugate movement of eyes; lateral, of course, but upward too. More of this later. Is there nystagmus?

(3) Hemiplegia; the tendon hammer may indicate only major lesions. Use the pronator test; the patient extends his supinated arms in front of him, and closes his eyes. Unilateral pronation is a good minimal sign of weakness; falling away of the arm may mean the same, or a sensory defect; tremor may be cerebellar.

Test fine movement – 'piano playing' with the fingers, wriggling of the toes. Test Hoffman's, superficial abdominals and plantars.

Then out with the tendon hammer, and complete the examination.

VITAL STATISTICS

70: 14: 120 may sound very inelegant as vital statistics, but are much healthier than 36: 23: 37 when pulse rate, respiration and systolic blood pressure are being considered. These figures are of great importance.

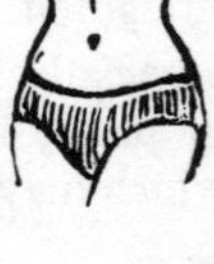

Especially if respiration is rapid, measure the rectal temperature.

CORRELATE AND DIAGNOSE

Don't ever accept a diagnosis of 'head injury' or of 'fractured skull' with a hotch-potch of mumbo-jumbo in the chart.

Work out the neurological lesions in relation to the known mechanism of injury and the scalp and skull findings.

The following examples refer to the primary injury and not to complications. The latter can be anticipated and diagnosed in the light of the primary assessment.

Case 1. Blunt trauma to scalp. No concussion. Left fronto-temporal scalp contusion with underlying linear fracture.

Right arm paresed, conjugate deviation of eyes to left.

Diagnosis: contusion of left frontal eyefield and arm area of cortex.

Case 2. Acceleration–deceleration injury with concussion. Right occipital bruise, no fracture.

Left face and arm paresed, stiff neck.

Regard as right frontal (sphenoidal ridge) contrecoup injury, probably laceration with subarachnoid haemorrhage.

Case 3. Acceleration–deceleration injury with concussion. Right parietal contusion.

Decerebrate rigidity plus complete right third nerve lesion.

Regard as avulsion of nerve from brainstem – primary third nerve and brainstem injury.

Case 4. Acceleration–deceleration injury with concussion. Frontal compound depressed fracture.

Left hemiplegia with gross spasticity, neurogenic hyperthermia.

Regard as upper brainstem injury.

Thus attempt accurate description of the lesion in every case.

RECOMMENDED FURTHER READING

Hooper, R. (1969). *Patterns of Acute Head Injury.* London: Edward Arnold

Part III
The Clinical Course

The initial examination gives information regarding the primary injury to the head; scalp, skull, nerves and brain. The subsequent clinical course allows assessment of the progress of the lesions sustained, and diagnosis of complications.

Consider the sea of consciousness.

The patient sails serenely on its surface (or gently immersed in it by the alcohol which will precipitate the next act) until the moment of injury.

If the injury be acceleration–deceleration in type, and concussion occurs, he is thrust suddenly into the depths. If he sinks too far, he hits the bottom and dies. Otherwise he stabilizes at some level or other.

This is immediate. There is no such thing as delayed concussion.

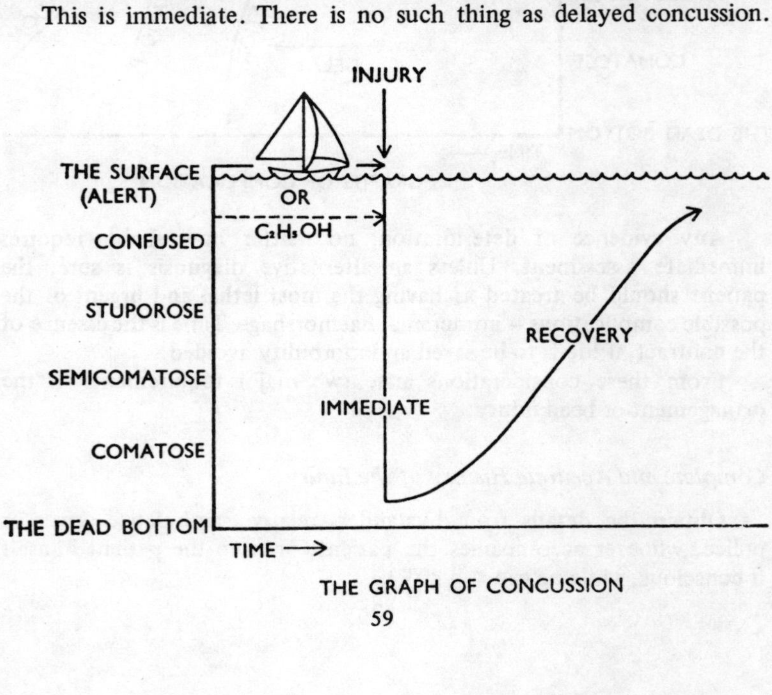

THE GRAPH OF CONCUSSION

He then tends to surface, for concussion tends to spontaneous recovery. He cannot deteriorate slowly or at an interval due to concussion.

This is the graph of concussion–an instantaneous plunge into unconsciousness, followed by stability and recovery.

Immediately the injury has been suffered the primary brain damage is complete, its neurological effects are maximal (though possibly obscured from the clinician by concussion), and its effect on consciousness is complete. *Therefore: any evidence of deterioration at an interval after injury is evidence of a complication of the injury*

This is the graph of complication; any downward trend in the post-injury course, any evidence of deterioration at an interval, means complication.

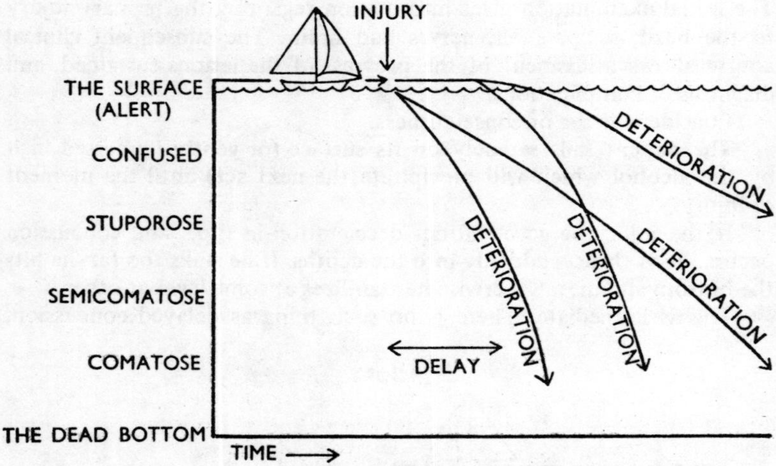

GRAPHS OF COMPLICATION

Any evidence of deterioration, no matter how slight, requires immediate assessment. Unless an alternative diagnosis is sure, the patient should be treated as having the most lethal and urgent of the possible complications – intracranial haemorrhage. Time is the essence of the contract, if life is to be saved and morbidity avoided.

From these considerations arise two major requirements in the management of head injury:

Complete and Accurate History of the Injury

Obtain the details from bystander, relative, ambulance driver or police, whoever accompanies the patient, or from the patient himself if conscious, while he can still give it!

The patient's state of consciousness between injury and arrival at hospital must be known if deterioration is to be detected early, otherwise only by further observation can the fact of progressive deterioration be determined.

The all too common 'motor car accident–alcohol–unconscious and can't give history' entry on a chart gives little information about the patient, but much about the doctor. He obviously neither appreciates nor cares about the nature of head injuries, and he is completely neglectful of his duty to the patient.

Full Observation as the Basis of Detection of Complications

The observations to be made are of state of consciousness, pupil size and reaction, pulse rate, systolic blood pressure, respiratory rate, and temperature when indicated.

Half-hourly is a routine frequency which may be increased when rapid change is occurring or anticipated, decreased when stability is achieved.

The clinical state after injury is never static. Recognize that changes may be occurring rapidly. Observe carefully and routinely in order to detect complications in time for useful treatment.

9—Acute Space-occupying Haematoma

'I am in blood
Stepp'd in so far that, should I wade no more,
Returning were as tedious as go o'er'.
Macbeth, Act III, Scene IV

Acute space-occupying haematomata (extradural, subdural or intracerebral) are the most dramatic of all complications of head injury. There is no substitute for early detection. The mortality and morbidity rate is directly proportional to the time wasted by unobservant or careless medical and nursing staff!

How do they present? Symptoms (in the conscious) and signs fall into three groups:

(1) Local effects of pressure upon or destruction of brain.
(2) General pressure effects.
(3) Signs of cerebral distortion.

Note that these signs are much the same whether the haematoma be extradural, subdural or intracerebral in site. Differentiation depends upon assessment of the proportions of various signs and correlation with the history and the scalp and skull evidence, as will be demonstrated.

LOCAL SIGNS

Hemiplegia or monoplegia, visual field loss, conjugate deviation of the eyes, sensory loss, cerebellar signs and so on, *developing at an interval after injury,* indicate a progressive lesion pressing upon or destroying the appropriate part of the brain.

But note that these signs may never appear; deep unconsciousness may mask them, or silent areas of brain may be involved.

Punter's Corner

Form Guide to Selection of Likely Starters

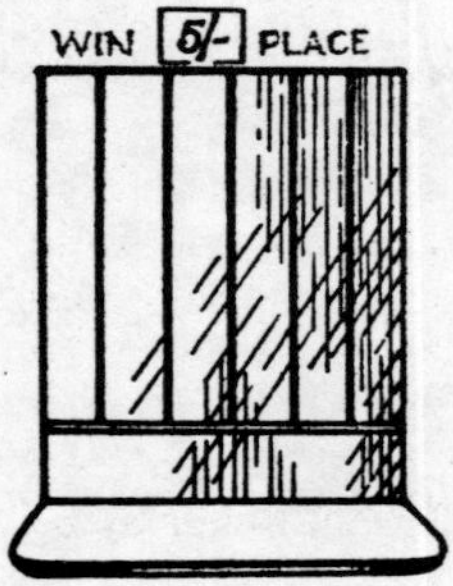

(1) Intracerebral haematoma tends to be discretely selective of particular cerebral functions.

(2) Subdural or extradural haematoma, on the cerebral surface, tend rather to produce a full hemiplegia and are less likely to cause 'intracerebral' phenomena, such as hemianopia or aphasia.

GENERAL PRESSURE EFFECTS

Headache is the leading symptom in this group. Many patients have headache after injury, but complaint of excessive headache and especially of increasing headache, should suggest rising pressure. The other leading possibility is continued subarachnoid bleeding.

Headache alone may lead to the diagnosis with only minimal supporting signs.

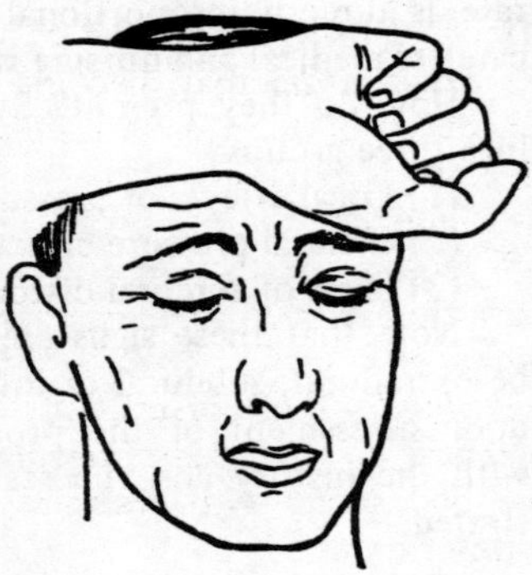

Restlessness may be evidence of headache, as may ***irritability*** in the less conscious patient. Increasing restlessness must be studied with care; it may be due to bladder filling or some other cause, but it may be the earliest sign of rising intracranial pressure.

Vital Statistics. Circulation and respiration are likely to be disturbed. Almost pathetic reliance has been placed upon certain particular changes as diagnostic of particular lesions, but the changes are quite non-specific.

The first effect of rising pressure upon the circulatory and respiratory centres is to stimulate them. Stimulation later gives way to depression, which progresses to paralysis. (This, of course, is the sequence of effects of almost any innovation, be it New Year's resolution or Town Planning.)

Respiration

Stimulation of the respiratory centre results in deepening of respiration without change in rate. Later, the respiratory rate may increase as discussed under hypothalamic and brainstem effects, but usually respiratory depression supervenes and results in progressive slowing.

Bradypnoea may be associated with increasingly shallow respiration, or apneustic gasping may occur. During the stage of depression there may be Cheyne Stokes respiration, a dysrhythmia demonstrating alternating stimulation and depression. This has been considered by many to be an ominous sign of compression, but remember that normal babies may exhibit it when going to sleep, as may patients with cardiac failure. All it means is that the respiratory centre is unstable and again time may be short.

Circulation

The circulatory centre has two dominant tones, vagal cardioinhibition and sympathetic vasoconstriction. Stimulation increases the effects of these so that the pulse slows and the blood pressure rises.

Bradycardia may become extreme, with the pulse rate as low as 35 per minute. (Should this persist, it may be wise to administer atropine to paralyse the vagus.)

Sinus arrhythmia may increase at the same time, and this increase is a most suggestive sign of circulatory centre stimulation. Rarely other arrhythmias may appear; pulsus alternans, and doubling and halving of the pulse rate.

Blood pressure rise affects the systolic much more than the diastolic pressure, so that pulse pressure increases, sometimes to the extent that the bed rocks with each heartbeat. This bed-rocking sign seems of serious moment.

As stimulation gives way to depression the pulse rate rises and blood pressure falls until circulatory failure supervenes.

Thus bradycardia and hypertension, quoted as classical signs of extradural haematoma, are but early evidence of circulatory centre stimulation.

They may not occur at all, or so briefly that they are missed between successive observations of the patient.

If they occur they are good evidence of progressive lesion, and particularly of rising intracranial pressure.

If they do not occur, or are missed, the first changes seen will be tachycardia and hypotension. These do not exclude a space-occupying haematoma, but indicate that it is already later than you think;

circulatory paralysis is imminent. When the graph of blood pressure in millimetres of mercury systolic crosses the pulse rate in beats per minute, the cross of death is drawn. Diagnose before this happens; waste no time in its presence.

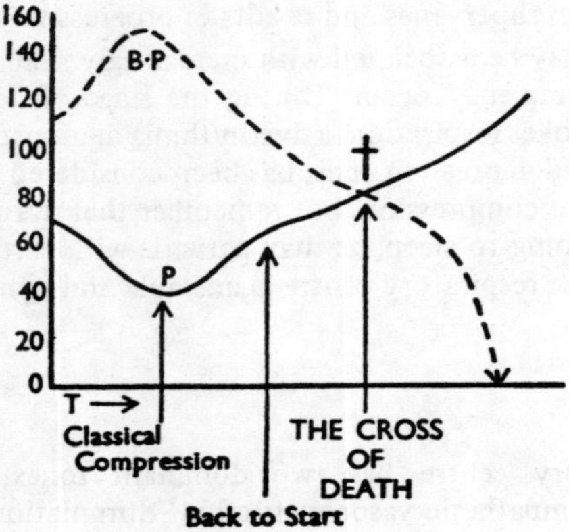

Early return of pulse rate towards normal when a haematoma is evacuated is a most useful indication of prognosis. Failure to improve spells impending disaster.

Increasing Unconsciousness

Increasing unconsciousness is the sign which is important above all others.

Any evidence of deterioration at an interval after injury is sufficient ground for suspicion. *Do not* await full coma, but note changes of a single step in the list of consciousness suggested earlier.

Lucid Interval

The importance of a lucid interval has been overstressed. When the patient, after concussion, regains full consciousness only to lapse again into coma, we have the most dramatic demonstration of deterioration at an interval. But the significance of deterioration is the same whether consciousness is regained before it or not; it means a complication of the injury.

Note. It should be one's object to operate upon the patient while he is still lucid, and before deepening coma imperils his life and raises morbidity.

ACUTE SPACE-OCCUPYING HAEMATOMA

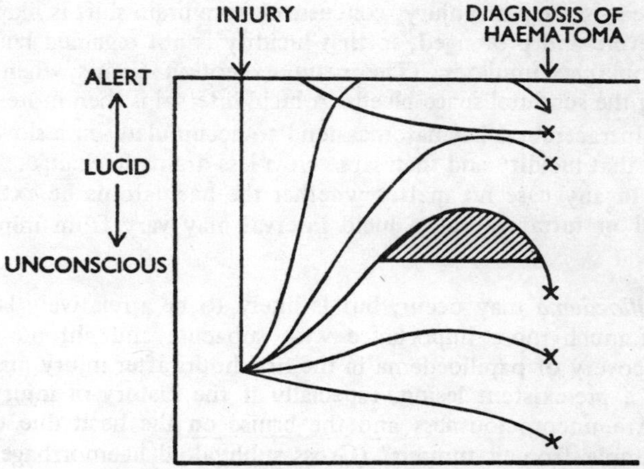

CLINICAL COURSES TO DIAGNOSIS

CLASSICAL LUCID INTERVAL (CROSS HATCHED) IS UNCOMMON

When patients with extradural haematoma are operated upon while conscious, the mortality rate is less than 5 per cent.

When patients are deeply semicomatose with fixed dilated pupils, the mortality rate approaches 75 per cent, and morbidity in the remainder is high.

Very often the difference between these groups is to be measured in terms of medical and nursing ignorance, ineptitude, procrastination and neglect.

Punters' Corner

Form Guide to Starters in the Lucid Stakes

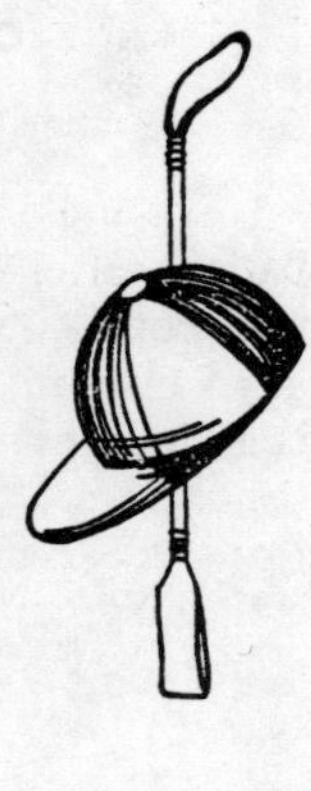

(1) Lucid interval is quoted as a classical sign of extradural haemorrhage, but it occurs in only 30 per cent of patients with this lesion.

(2) Extradural haemorrhage tends to occur in relatively less severe injuries than subdural; thus it is more likely that the patient will regain consciousness from initial concussion to produce a lucid interval.

(3) Subdural haematoma is most common as the result of a cerebral laceration from the sphenoidal

ridge area. In such an injury, concussion from brain shift is likely to be more severe and prolonged, so that lucidity is not regained before the haematoma accumulates. (The main exception occurs when a vein bridging the subdural space bleeds. A lucid interval is then more likely.)

(4) Intracerebral haematomas tend to accumulate on a slower time base, so that lucidity and then lapse are a less dramatic change.

(5) In any case no matter whether the haematoma be extradural, subdural or intracerebral, a lucid interval may vary from minutes to days.

Papilloedema may occur, but is likely to be a relatively late sign. It is of much more importance with subacute and chronic lesions. The discovery of papilloedema in the first hours after injury makes one suspect a pre-existent lesion, especially if the history of injury is not clear. Are unconsciousness and the bruise on the head due to a fit, for example from a tumour? (Gross subhyaloid haemorrhage always suggests cerebral aneurysm.)

SIGNS OF CEREBRAL DISTORTION

As a haematoma expands, it displaces and distorts the brain. Two particular levels are especially prone to damage by distortion—the

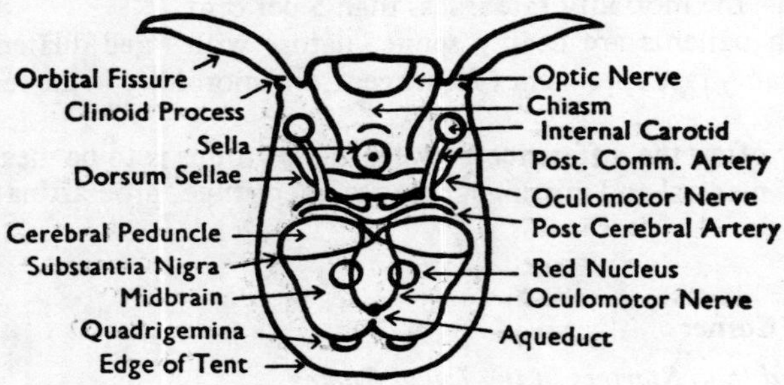

THE BRAINSTEM IS THE DONKEY

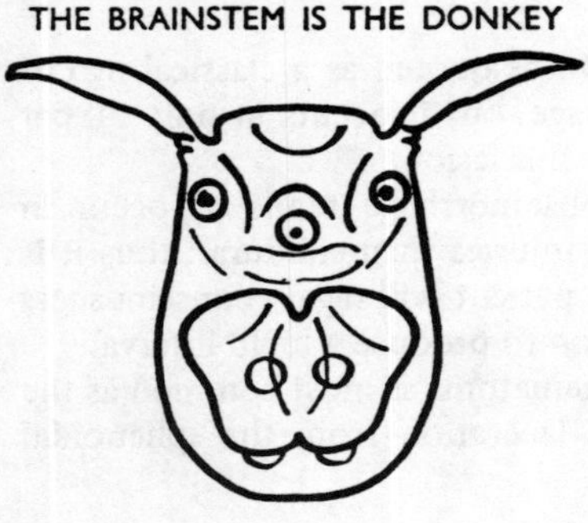

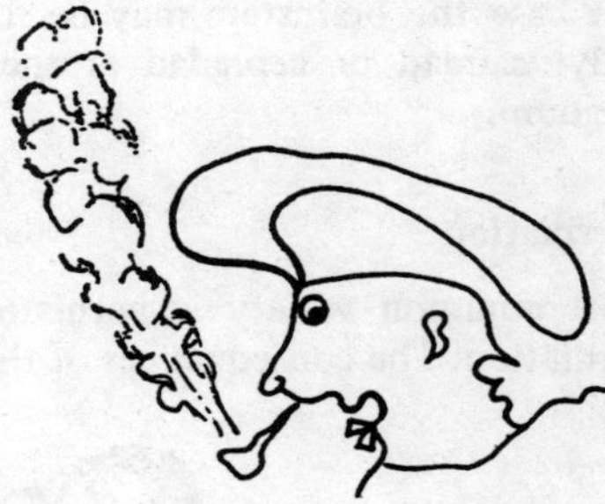

THE ACADEMIC

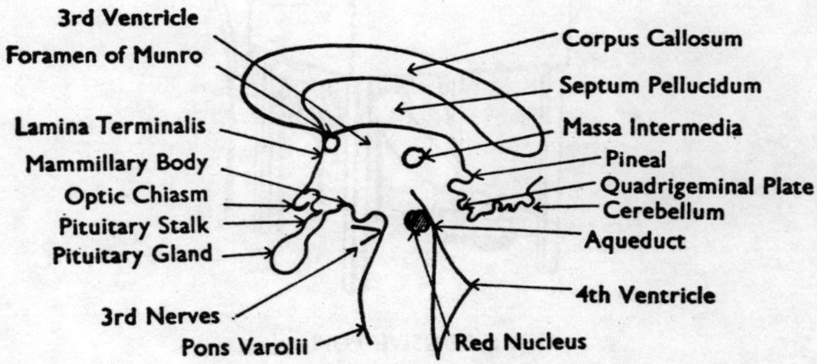

THE PRACTICAL

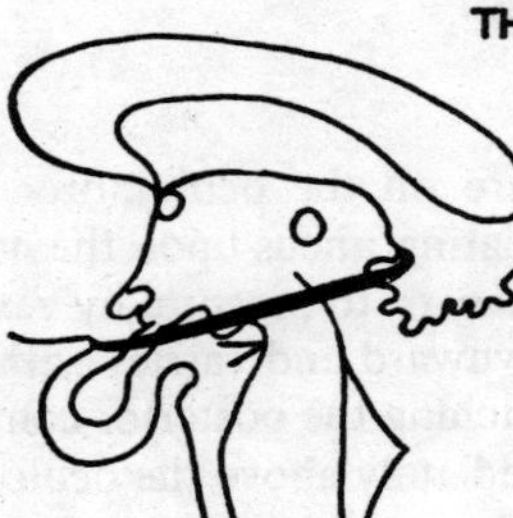

THE TENTORIUM

midbrain at the level of the tentorium cerebelli, and the medulla at the level of the foramen magnum. At either level a 'pressure cone' may develop by the herniation of cerebral structures beside the brainstem.

At tentorial level this is likely to involve the uncinate processes of the temporal lobes if the pressure is from above, or the cerebellar hemispheres if the pressure if from below.

At the foramen magnum, the cerebellar tonsils may be herniated into the cervical spinal canal.

In either case the brainstem may be shifted both transversely and longitudinally, caudad or cephalad at the tentorium, caudad at the foramen magnum.

Tentorial Herniation

The most common variety is herniation from above, also called uncinate herniation. The consequences of this are as follows.

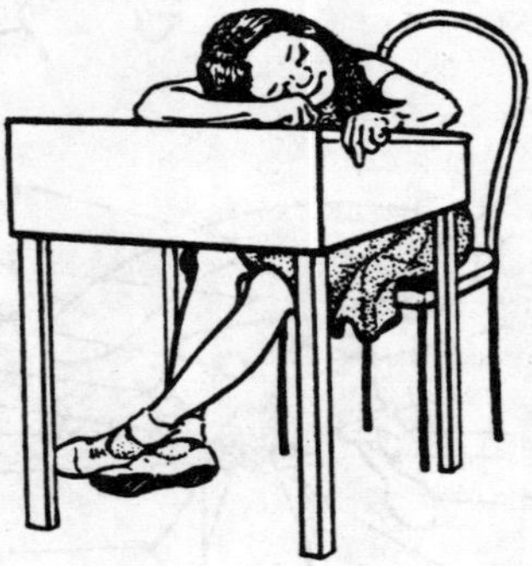

UNRESPONSIVE PUPIL

Pupil Effects

Pupillary changes are due to pressure on the oculomotor nerve. This may be due to pressure of the herniating uncus upon the nerve in the case of anteriorly situated haematomas, or to pressure by vessels in other cases. The brainstem is pushed downward and carries with it the basilar and posterior cerebral arteries, stretching the posterior communicating artery. These latter vessels pass immediately above the oculomotor nerve at its origin from the midbrain, and may then compress its upper surface. (The pressure on the posterior cerebral artery, and its attenuation by stretching, may cause occipital infarction.)

Upon the upper surface of the oculomotor nerve run the parasympathetic pupilloconstrictor fibres.

The first effect of pressure is stimulation, so that the pupil constricts —a transitory stage that may be missed. Then paralysis supervenes, and the pupil progressively dilates and loses its reaction to light. Thus the fixed dilated pupil.

Note. (1) The dilated pupil is almost invariably on the side of the lesion, but in the early stages the smaller pupil may be the abnormal one. (When the fixed dilated pupil is contralateral to a haematoma, it is probably due to primary third nerve damage.)

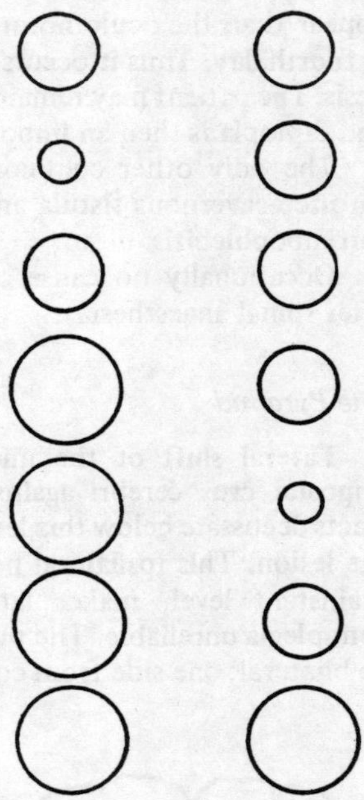

(2) The change is progressive, and once dilatation starts it usually continues uninterrupted. However, a small bleed may cause dilatation of the pupil which then subsides as the haematoma is accommodated. Further bleeding occurring later causes fresh dilatation.

(3) The fluctuating pupil is more likely to be due to brainstem dysfunction.

(4) The external ocular musculature is rarely involved unless the process occurs very slowly, over a period of days. This is one of the distinguishing features from primary third nerve damage; but a complete third nerve lesion may be produced occasionally by compression when the process occurs with extreme rapidity in the course of a few minutes.

(5) As distortion continues, the contralateral third nerve may also be involved with pupillary constriction and then dilatation. Bilateral fixed dilated pupils carry an extremely poor prognosis. Don't wait this late!

The uncus was pushed through the tent,
The oculomotor was bent,
The pupil constricted and then it dilated,
The other one followed–and he was cremated!

(6) The significant change is one that occurs at an interval after injury. If the pupil is dilated very early after the injury, and especially if strabismus is present, primary injury to the nerve is probable.

The Abducens

The sixth nerve may be similarly involved by herniation, giving rise to a delayed strabismus due to lateral rectus palsy. This condition is more often seen with posteriorly situated lesions, or with reversed tentorial coning from posterior fossa haematomas. It usually takes longer to appear than the oculomotor lesion, and is not common before the third or fourth day. Thus it occurs with lesions accumulating on a slower time basis. The patient may remain conscious while the abducens palsy occurs, and diplopia is then an important symptom.

The only other common causes of delayed sixth nerve lesion are carotico-cavernous fistula and, rarely, involvement by superior petrosal thrombophlebitis.

Occasionally no cause can be found (compare lateral rectus palsy after spinal anaesthesia).

The Pyramid

Lateral shift of the midbrain may be sufficient to compress the opposite crus cerebri against the tentorial edge. Since the pyramidal tracts decussate below this level, there results a hemiplegia on the side of the lesion. This ipsilateral hemiplegia, commonly spastic because of its brainstem level, makes lateralization of the lesion on grounds of hemiplegia unreliable. The pupil is a much better guide. Hemiplegia may be bilateral; one side from cortical level, the other from brainstem.

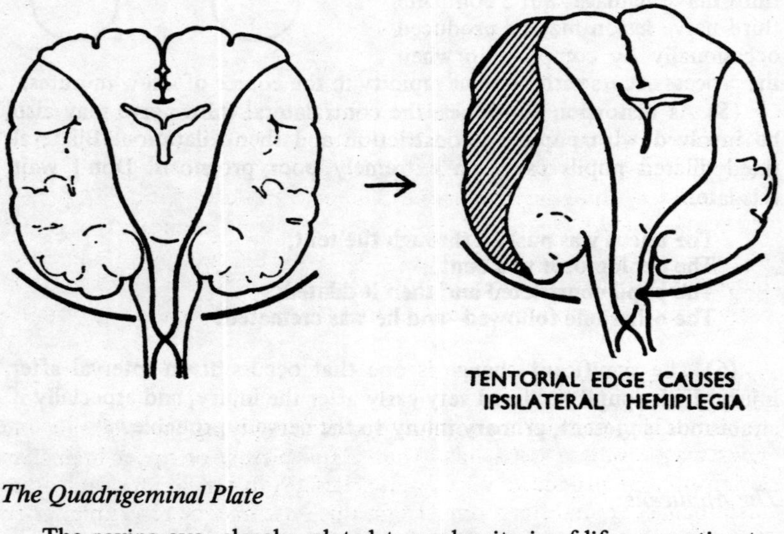

TENTORIAL EDGE CAUSES IPSILATERAL HEMIPLEGIA

The Quadrigeminal Plate

The roving eye, closely related to such criteria of life as reaction to simulus and reproduction, is a valuable sign of viability.

If the eyes are roving, then the quadrigeminal plate is still functioning.

In general, if cerebral distortion is such that unconsciousness (interference with the brainstem reticular formation) and a dilated pupil have resulted, the quadrigeminal plate will also be paralysed by pressure and the eyes will be stationary.

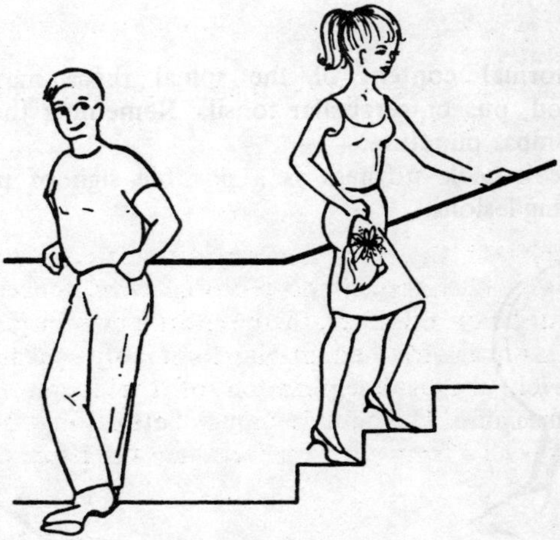

ROVING EYE

If the eyes are roving or can be made to rove conjugately by rolling the head of the patient when unconscious, an alternative explanation of loss of consciousness (e.g., recent epilepsy) or of a fixed dilated pupil (e.g., primary third nerve injury) should be considered strongly.

With slowly forming collections above the tentorium the first effect on the quadrigeminal plate may be to cause loss of upward conjugate movement of the eyes (compare pinealoma), and this may be a valuable early sign of distortion in lesions such as chronic subdural haematoma.

Midbrain and Pons

Stretching of small perforating arteries supplying the midbrain and pons may result in ischaemia. Thus a full picture of upper brainstem lesion may be produced; decerebrate rigidity, hyperthermia, and other disturbances of vital function. At first this state may be reversible, when only ischaemia is present, but irreversible changes rapidly follow as definitive damage from infarction and haemorrhage supervenes.

It is these changes that are responsible for much of the mortality and crippling morbidity caused by intracranial haematoma.

The Medullary Cone

Tonsillar herniation through the foramen magnum may produce few signs, but the following should be noted:

Stiff Neck

Any abnormal content of the spinal theca may cause neck stiffness–blood, pus or cerebellar tonsils. Remember the latter before performing lumbar puncture.

Always seek neck stiffness as a possible sign of posterior fossa space-occupying lesions.

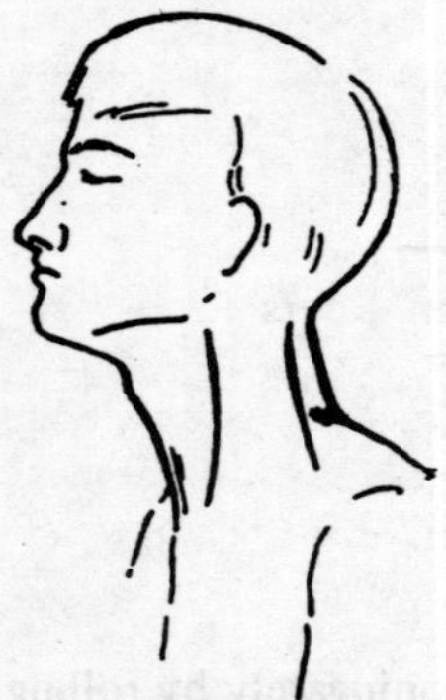

STIFF NECK

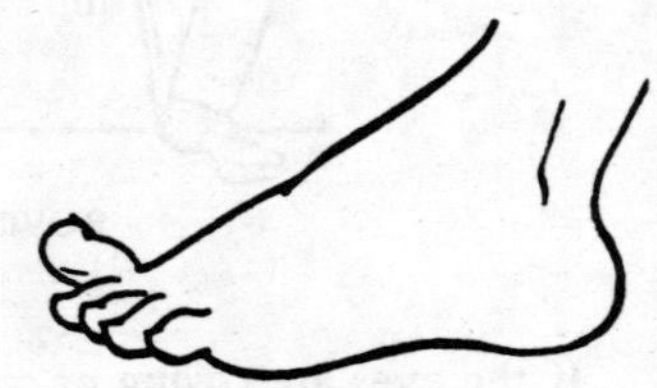

TOE UP

Pyramidal Signs

Pyramidal signs may appear due to compression of the medulla by the tonsils, or against the edge of the foramen magnum. A previously normal plantar response which becomes abnormal may be the sole neurological sign exhibited by posterior fossa extradural haematoma.

Cerebellar Signs

Cerebellar signs are conspicuously absent with posterior fossa extradural haematoma except when it evolves slowly. However, when a posterior fossa extradural haematoma first presents on the seventh to tenth day, it may do so with all the signs suggestive of a cerebellar tumour.

Posterior fossa subdural haematoma, or cerebellar laceration and intracerebellar haematoma, produce cerebellar signs much more readily.

Medullary Failure

This may occur suddenly.

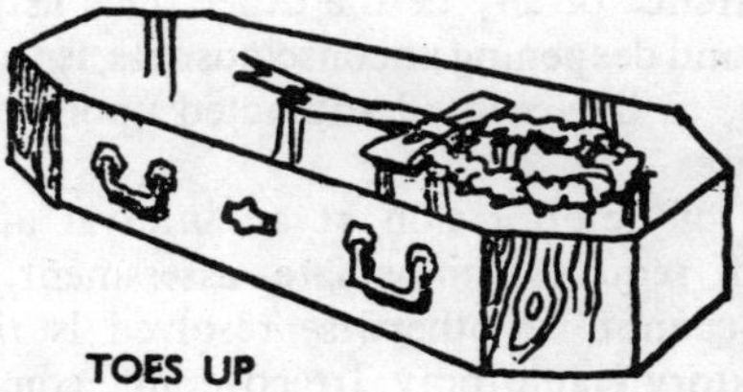

Its features are flaccidity (contrast spasticity with lesions above the vestibular nuclei), respiratory collapse and circulatory failure.

Note that respiration, which is dependent upon an intact respiratory centre and cervical cord, may cease while circulation is maintained by cardiac action without central control.

Circulation may continue for minutes or even hours after final apnoea.

Once respiration ceases there is little hope of rescue of patients with supratentorial lesions. Even if respiration should start again, the cerebral cortex is usually irreparably damaged by high supratentorial pressure. The respiratory centre can be restarted after up to thirty minutes of anoxia, the cortex survives only four to five minutes. However, immediate artificial respiration may dispel hypercapnia and hypoxia, and permit recovery if urgent surgical action follows.

With posterior fossa lesions, immediate craniotomy after apnoea may be successful, for the major pressure has been in the posterior fossa, sparing the cerebral cortex.

SUMMARY

This chapter seems to have presented a rather indigestable account of possible events. Therefore note the following points of importance.

(1) The full classical picture described is a rarity—it will occur in only 30 per cent of extradural haematomas, less of subdural and intracerebral.

(2) If you wait for the full classical picture, you wait for death, or irreversible morbidity.

(3) The only uniformly reliable symptoms and signs are increasing headache and irritability in the conscious, deepening unconsciousness in the unconscious.

(4) The occurrence of any of the other signs listed above, with or without headache and deepening unconsciousness, is to be regarded as an undeserved bonus, to be accepted and acted upon with gratitude. But don't expect bonuses.

(5) Any sign of deterioration at an interval after injury means complication and requires immediate assessment. Suspicion of a haematoma that cannot be otherwise resolved is *the* indication for immediate exploratory craniotomy. Irrecoverable complications may be imminent.

'Will you walk a little faster?',
Said the surgeon to the nurse,
'There's the Reaper close behind me
And he's followed by the hearse'.

Punter's Corner

Guide to All Starters in the Haematoma Handicap

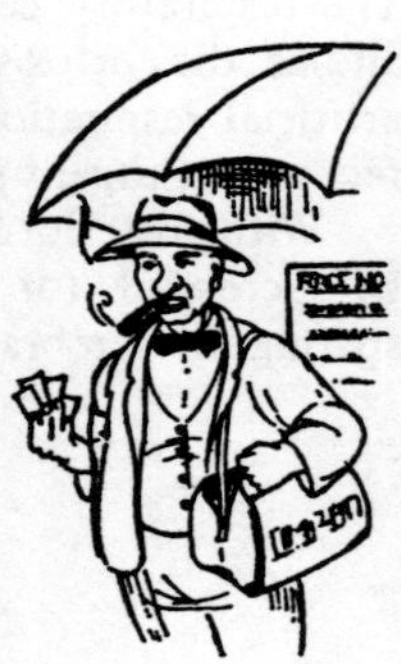

Having diagnosed a space-occupying haematoma, which lesion will you back? At best you can assess probabilities, and quote the odds.

(1) If the haematoma is contralateral to the skull trauma, it is not extradural.

(2) If the signs place the haematoma far from the site of trauma, it is not extradural.

(3) The more 'classical' the story, lucid interval and all, the more likely is the haematoma to be extradural.

(4) The less neurological signs immediately after trauma, the less likely is subdural haematoma.

(5) The more precisely localizable the lesion neurologically, the more likely it is to be intracerebral.

(6) Anterior fossa, occipital and posterior fossa lesions produce fewest signs to warn of impending disaster.

(7) If in doubt, back all starters in this race. Drill at the site of trauma, and at the site of subdural haematoma bilaterally if necessary.

There is no substitute for early diagnosis and minimal time loss. Even if life is saved, wasted time may mean irreparable morbidity.

ACUTE SPACE-OCCUPYING HAEMATOMA

Suspicion of an extradural haematoma plus clinical or radiological evidence of a fracture crossing the course of a vessel is an absolute indication for immediate craniotomy.

Recognize the possibility.
Observe the patient.
Diagnose any deterioration.
Act!

RECOMMENDED FURTHER READING

Jamieson, K.G. and Yelland, J.D.N. (1968). 'Extradural Haematoma'. *J. Neurosurg.* **29**, 13

McKissock, W., Richardson, A. and Bloom, W.H. (1960). 'Subdural Haematoma'. *Lancet* **1**, 1365

10—Inoperable Haemorrhage and Oedema

Deterioration at an interval always means that a complication has occurred, and operable, remediable lesions must be thought of first.

But all that glisters is not gold; some patients deteriorate because their injuries are complicated by continuing inoperable haemorrhage and oedema.

The problem is how to pick them. To operate or not to operate, that is the question.

The Nature of the Complication

When any cerebral vessel, large or small, has been injured (on the surface by skull ridges or in the depths by shearing stress) it may continue to bleed. Areas of contusion may become oedematous, resulting in cellular anoxia and dysfunction.

If this haemorrhage and oedema occur in relation to vital areas, as in primary brainstem or hypothalamic injury, then death may occur rapidly.

If the haemorrhage and oedema occur locally in non-vital areas, then localized space-occupying lesions may occur as considered earlier.

When they occur in widespread fashion throughout the brain, non-specific and inoperable deterioration may occur.

The clue is the clinical course. A full history is vital to diagnosis.

Consider the following generalizations:

(1) When death is immediate, brain injury is usually found to be overwhelmingly severe. (But note that death may occur from concussion without any macroscopic evidence of brain injury.)

(2) When the injury appears to have been relatively minor (from the point of view of cerebral symptoms and signs), deterioration is most likely due to extradural haemorrhage from injury to the coverings. (But

note that veins may be torn or silent areas lacerated without neurological sign, so that subdural haemorrhage can be the cause.)

(3) The more severe the signs of cerebral injury initially, the more likely are lacerations, surface and depth shearing, to have occurred. Thus subdural and intracerebral haematomas are more likely. (But note that injury to the coverings coexists so that extradural haematoma may still occur.)

(4) The more profound and severe the signs of cerebral damage initially, the more likely is the damage to be widespread, and the more likely is the complication of haemorrhage and oedema to be multicentric or generalized, and inoperable. (But note that isolated surface haemorrhage could still occur.)

(5) The longer the patient survives before deterioration occurs, the less likely is irrecoverable cerebral damage and widespread haemorrhage and oedema. (But note that patients may survive irrecoverable damage for months or years.)

(6) If the patient starts to improve before deterioration, then local complication of local damage is more likely than general inoperable haemorrhage and oedema.

So much for the general form guide. In each individual instance, assess the odds.

Unlikely Starters

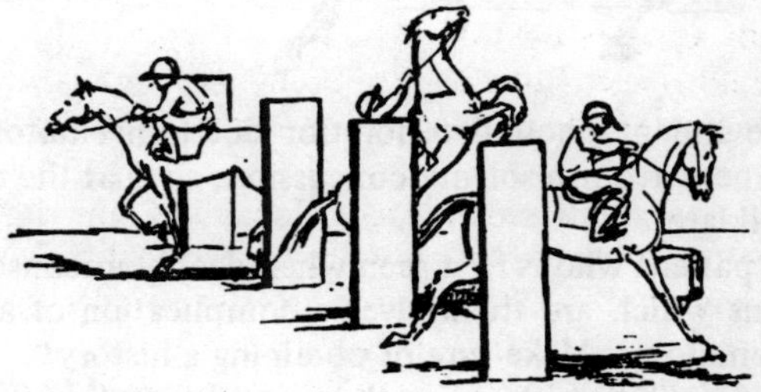

The patient who is clearly moribund from the moment of injury and dies rapidly.

The patient with gross decerebrate spasms soon after injury who never rallies, but fades out gradually.

The patient who shows a steady non-specific down-hill course from an initially serious state.

Favoured Candidates

Those who deteriorate from an initially mild or only moderately severe injury.

Those who improve from a serious injury, or at least stabilize for a period, and then deteriorate.

Those who have scalp and skull signs or a clinical course suggestive of a focal lesion.

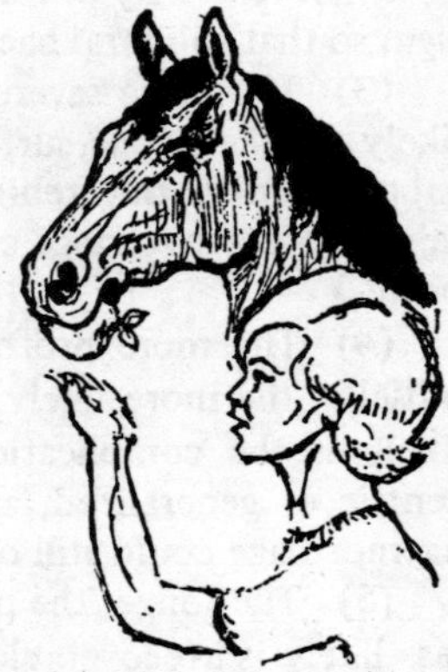

The Dark Horse

This is the worry, but he is not common. This is the patient who deteriorates rapidly, often with a massive subdural haematoma, from an initially satisfactory state.

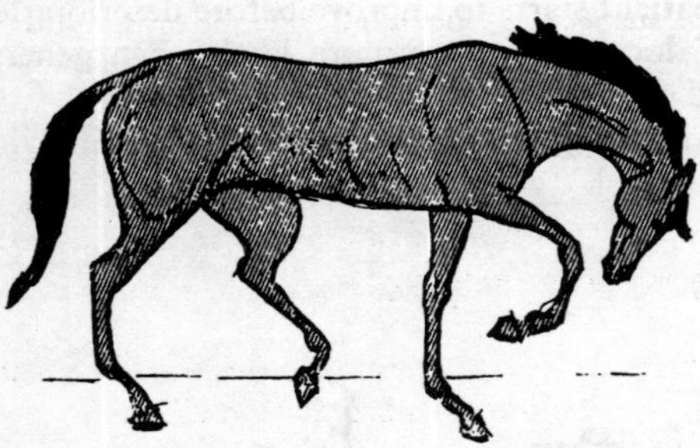

This is the patient whose deterioration due to haematoma coincides with improvement from resolving concussion, so that the deterioration is masked until late.

This is the patient who is first seen when deeply unconscious or with brainstem signs which are themselves a complication of a local space-occupying haematoma. Make sure of obtaining a history!

This is the patient with more than one haematoma, each and all operable and remediable, but difficult to detect because of their multiplicity.

Ill-advice to Beginners

This, culled from standard textbooks, includes:

(1) *Setting a time limit.* It has been said that one should never operate earlier than four hours after injury. Some element of truth may

be found here, for most space-occupying haematomata take longer than this to form. But some perfectly remediable lesions will cause death faster than this.

Don't watch the clock and delay, watch the patient and act!

(2) *Awaiting the classical indication.* This manoeuvre (procrastination until action is forced) is rewarded by the classical results, which are excessively bad. Most cases will not be classical; recognize early deterioration, assess urgently, and act.

THE TRUE SITUATION

When deterioration starts it usually progresses to death unless remedial action is taken.

If you do nothing, the patient will probably die.

If you drill inspection holes at the appropriate sites you will: (*i*) find any remediable lesion; or (*ii*) do no harm.

If you can suspect a localized haematoma, you must operate.

Only with increasing experience will you learn when operation is futile or unnecessary.

Not the greater your experience, the more operations you perform, *but* the less your experience, the more operations you must perform.

The smaller the proportion of negative craniotomies, the more remediable lesions you are missing.

'Diseases desperate grown, by desperate measures
are relieved, or not at all.'

NON-OPERATIVE TREATMENT

When a decision is made that operation has nothing to offer a patient, it is more necessary than ever that non-operative care of the patient should be conducted with extreme care.

In a later chapter we shall discuss the details of care designed to reduce or prevent haemorrhage and oedema. Cerebral venous congestion is the greatest danger to such a patient, and may be alleviated by careful attention to posture and respiration.

It is most important to recognize that non-operative care in any case of head injury is at least as important as treatment by operation.

Part IV of this book deals with general care, but here specific reference may be made to various measures which may be used in an endeavour to control cerebral oedema and raised pressure.

Osmotic Diuretic Agents

The most commonly used agents in this group are mannitol and fructose, urea now being largely outmoded. Mannitol in particular may be given in an endeavour to dehydrate the brain to reduce cerebral oedema and to lower raised intracranial pressure. Great caution is necessary in this usage.

Mannitol is excellent for shrinking normal brain to improve exposure, but is less effective in damaged brain with a disturbed blood-brain barrier. Further, any dramatic reduction in cerebral volume may precipitate haemorrhage – new or recurrent – from cerebral lacerations or torn veins. Its use in head injury should be restricted to:

(*i*) reduction of pressure while preparations for surgery are made in critical cases;

(*ii*) control of pressure during transfer of a patient; and

(*iii*) selective use in post-operative care.

Beware of electrolyte disturbances. Mannitol may produce hyponatremia and cerebral oedema.

Dexamethasone

Administration of dexamethasone in case of cerebral oedema about tumours is dramatically effective. Regrettably it is much less useful in the case of head injury, but some reasonable case may be made for its usage in patients with severe brainstem injury although there is as yet no definite evidence as to its efficacy.

Induced Hypothermia

Reference has already been made to the cooling of patients with neurogenic hyperthermia and of patients with brainstem spasms. Experience would now suggest that induced hypothermia beyond control of pyrexia is not effective in management of the general range of head injuries.

Hyper-ventilation and Controlled Ventilation

Reference will be made to these matters in the section on respiration.

Cerebral Blood Flow

Loss of auto-regulation of the cerebral circulation with gross increase in cerebral blood flow is common in severe injury. No regimem for management of this problem has yet been established.

RECOMMENDED FURTHER READING

Galicich, J.H. and French, L.A. (1961). 'Use of Dexamethasone in the Treatment of Cerebral Oedema Resulting from Brain Tumours and Surgery'. *Am. Practnr. Dig. Treat.* **12**, 169

Rowbotham, G.F. (1949). *Acute Injuries of the Head*, 3rd ed. Edinburgh: Livingstone

Shenkin, H.A., Goluboff, B. and Haft, H. (1962). 'The Use of Mannitol for the Reduction of Intracranial Pressure in Intracranial Surgery'. *J. Neurosurg.* **19**, 897

11—Delayed Haematoma and Hygroma

So far we have considered chiefly the events of the first few hours or days after injury, and the acute complications that occur therein. So much for the sprinters, though some extradural haematomata may last into the middle distance of seven to ten days or more.

We must now consider the stayers that appear in the longer run of up to six weeks or more after the injury. These are:

Subacute and chronic subdural haematoma.

Subdural 'hygroma'.

'Spatapoplexie traumatische'.

SUBACUTE AND CHRONIC SUBDURAL HAEMATOMA

These haematomata are quite different from those considered earlier, most of which arose from cerebral lacerations in relation to the sphenoidal ridge area.

Subacute and especially chronic subdural haematomata usually occur high over the convexities of the hemispheres.

The Subacute Haematoma

This may arise by non-fatal persistence of an acute haematoma until late in the first week, or up to three weeks after injury. It is then sometimes clearly related to a cerebral laceration, but more often no causative laceration is found. Probably it arises from a vein avulsion injury.

The haematoma may occupy the whole subdural space of a hemicranium, and is usually relatively shallow (up to 2 cm deep), and mainly solid clot.

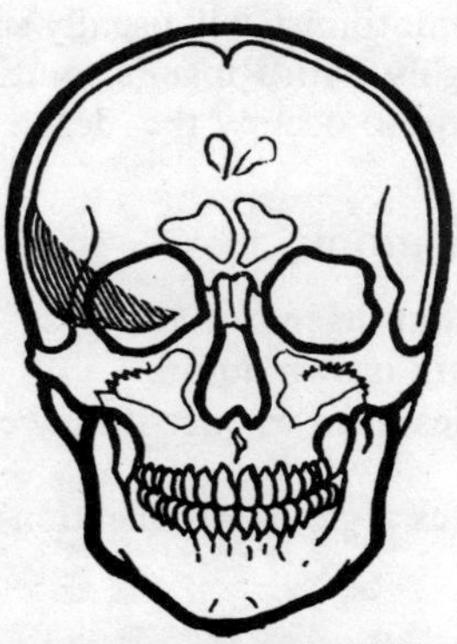

THE ACUTE SUBDURAL HAEMATOMA

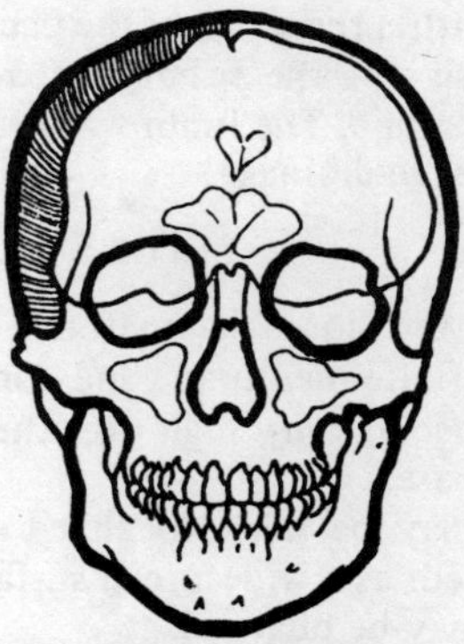

THE USUAL SUBACUTE SUBDURAL

Common features are:

(1) High pressure; severe headache, and papilloedema may occur.

(2) Localizing signs like those of acute haematomata, on a slower time base, are seen.

(3) False localizing signs; abducens palsy, paralysis of upward conjugate deviation, and ipsilateral hemiplegia are often found.

(4) Flattening of the cranial percussion note on the affected side is a useful sign.

Warning

This is one of the most unfriendly lesions met by the surgeon. Once it presents clinically, enforcing diagnostic endeavour, it rarely permits longevity sufficient for liquefaction of the haematoma to the 'chronic' state. Secondary brainstem haemorrhage occurs first.

Therefore, it must be removed whilst solid!

Procedure

A burrhole in the temporal fossa (as for acute subdural haematoma) will reveal solid clot.

The hole should then be enlarged to form a large subtemporal decompression through which clot can be removed by suction, by irrigation, and by dissection. If necessary the gloved finger may be used for dissection of the clot from the dura, but avoid tearing veins as they enter venous sinuses. In young people neurosurgeons often resort to an osteoplastic flap for this lesion, but a subtemporal decompression, much more within the scope of the occasional craniotomist, will usually suffice.

Wash out the subdural space thoroughly with Ringer's solution or normal saline. The brain will usually expand to occupy the 'dead space'.

Provide drainage!

The Chronic Haematoma

This is the liquid haematoma, the subdural 'haemorrhagic cyst', lined by a definite membrane and containing dark brown liquid.

It occurs *only* high over the convexities from whence it may extend to the base.

It may be fairly localized and deep (as a globular collection) or it may occur as a widespread surface film.

It may be bilateral.

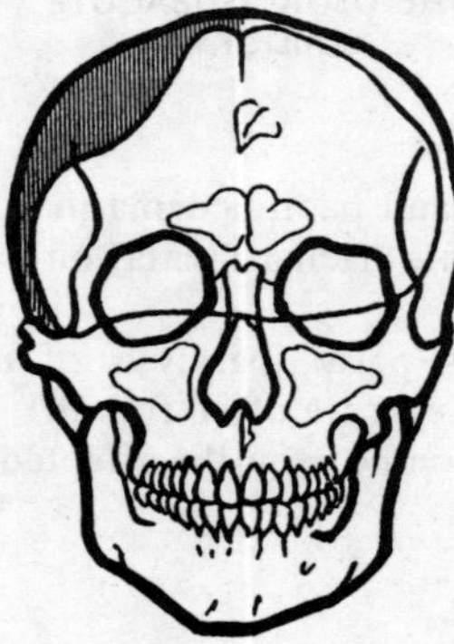

THE TYPICAL CHRONIC SUBDURAL

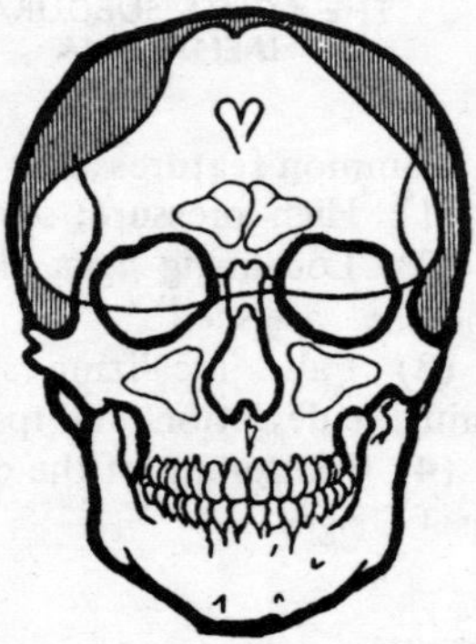

MAY BE BILATERAL

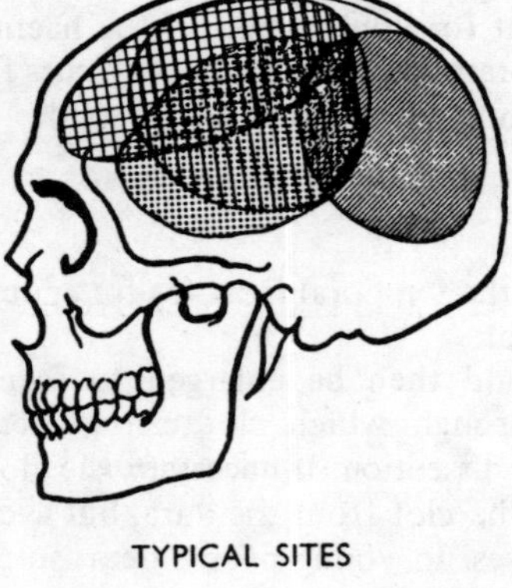

TYPICAL SITES

It presents usually three to six weeks after the injury. (Note especially this time relationship. Contrary to popular misconception, haematomas of longer standing than this – as seen from deposit of iron pigment in their walls – are now a rarity. The old pachymeningitis haemorrhagica has almost disappeared, along perhaps with the good old days of vitamin deficient diets and spirochaete spoilt pleasures.)

Common features are:

(1) Fluctuation in the state of consciousness. This is the sign *par excellence* of the chronic subdural haematoma. The patient is drowsy or even unrousable one day, conscious the next, only to lapse again, and so on. Such a story shouts 'Subdural'.

(2) Low pressure is often found – 30 or 40 mm only of cerebrospinal fluid pressure at lumbar puncture, while the fluid is commonly xanthochromic. Headache may not be complained of at all.

(3) Localizing features may be almost absent, though hemiplegia is usual – contra or ipsilateral. Upward conjugate gaze is often deficient, and the cranial percussion note may be flattened.

(4) False localizing signs are often seen, and in variety sufficient to mimic all manner of brainstem lesions to the deception of the very elect.

Warning

Many of these patients die with a diagnosis of 'stroke', especially cerebral thrombosis; yet it is one of the most readily treated and best prognosis lesions of all. Ask, 'Is this a stroke, or was he struck?'

Remember that the lesion may occur spontaneously, without trauma, or by rupture of an aneurysm into the subdural space. It is *the* lesion of alcoholics. Indeed, the following patients died of subdural haematoma:

An old man was found on the ground –
Some days he'd almost come round.
They stood and debated
While he fluctuated,
At P.M. a large clot was found.

A rather young alcoholic
Didn't wake up from a frolic;
'A surfeit of grog
Or a stroke', said the log –
'Thombotic or even embolic'.

An old girl as quaint as a fable
Would waken a little when able.
Carotid stenosis
Was one diagnosis –
You know what was found on the table!

An unconscious man was referred –
No story of how it occurred –
They said, 'It's a stroke
In this poor old bloke'.
Absurd – for he should have been burred!

Procedure

If you suspect the lesion, x-ray the skull. A single antero-posterior shot may show the pineal shift that indicates space-occupying lesion. Operate now or the brainstem may bleed before tomorrow!

Drill a high temporal burrhole. Dark dura invites the knife to expose the dark liquid that runs out easily.

Wash out thoroughly with saline or Ringer's solution until the washings are clear.

If the haematoma is extensive, drill a high posterior parietal hole, and wash out through and through.

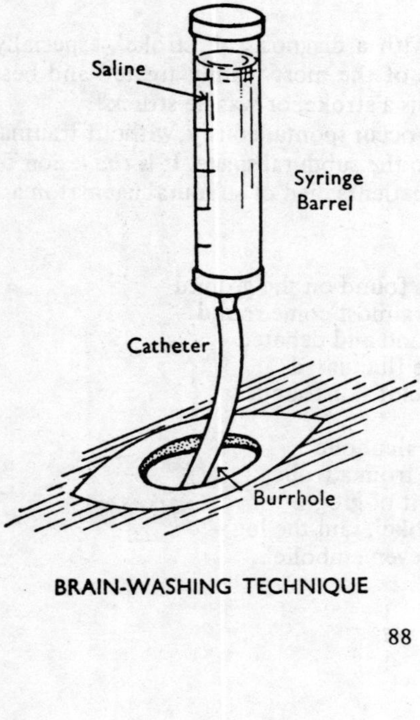

BRAIN-WASHING TECHNIQUE

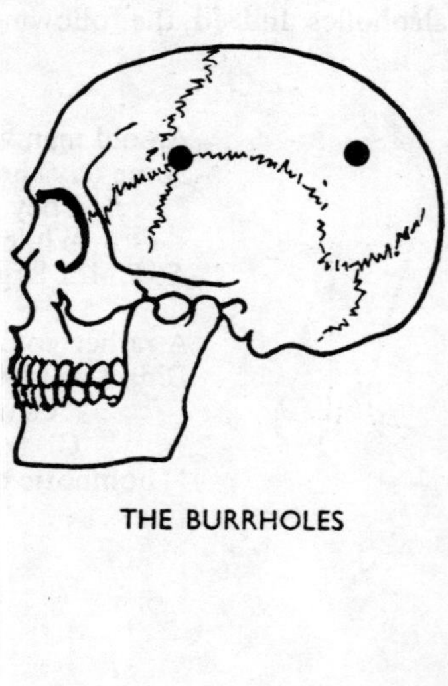

THE BURRHOLES

If the anterior hole shows no haematoma, drill the posterior one and look there.

Unless you are sure the lesion is unilateral (pineal shift is gross, or angiograms have been done), explore the other side.

Drain!

Problem Corner

The Brain Won't Come Up?

The lesion is a low pressure one because the brain is dehydrated, often with collapsed ventricles, and herniated through the tentorial hiatus.

Lumbar puncture the patient while the wound is open and inject, or preferably instil by gravity flow, Ringer's solution (saline will do) until normal lumbar pressure is achieved. Up to 100 ml or more may be needed. Watch the brain come up as the uncinate hernia is reduced like a cork from a bottle and the ventricles expand.

It used to be fashionable to speak of the mysterious 'low pressure syndrome' of continuing drowsiness and low cerebrospinal fluid pressure after operation. This was really unrelieved tentorial herniation, not seen since inflation with fluid has been practised.

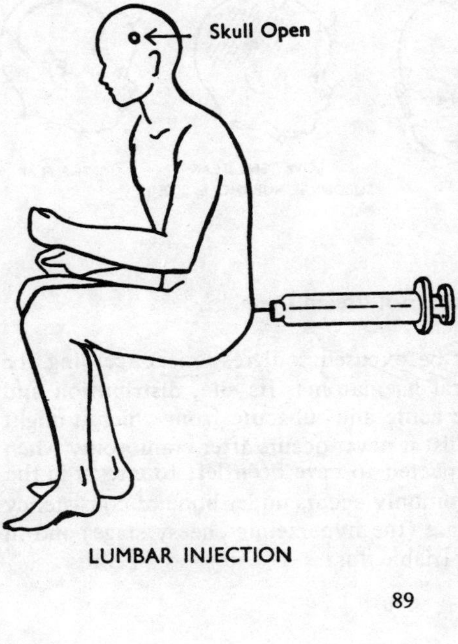

LUMBAR INJECTION

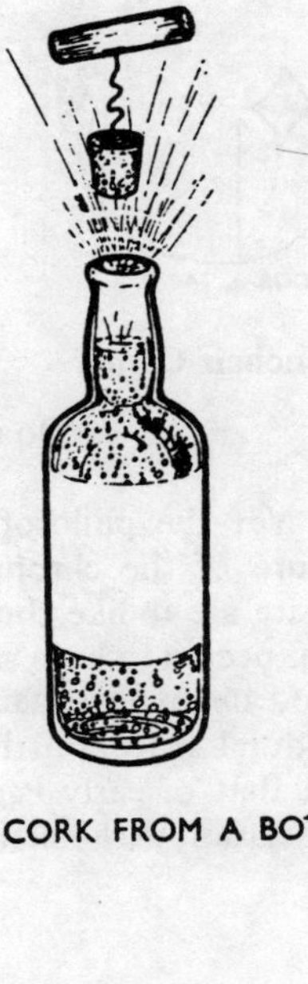

LIKE A CORK FROM A BOTTLE

The Post-operative Course is Unsatisfactory?

Consider the possibility of brainstem haemorrhage from prolonged distortion. Make sure the haematoma has not re-accumulated.

Special Note re Infants

Infantile birth trauma, from skull moulding during delivery, may result in subdural haematoma. The causative lesion is often a tentorial tear or avulsion of veins from its surface.

The acute lesion presents as an acute haematoma with tense fontanelle, depression of consciousness, disturbance of respiration (often with apnoeic periods), epileptic fits and hemiplegia. Needle the subdural space through the lateral angle of the fontanelle as a diagnostic procedure, drill a hole (remembering the possibly low site of origin) and wash out the clot.

The subacute lesion presents as a cause of enlarging head, with neurological signs.

The chronic lesion usually presents as 'failure to thrive'. An osteoplastic flap and excision of the membrane may be necessary if washing out through burrholes fails.

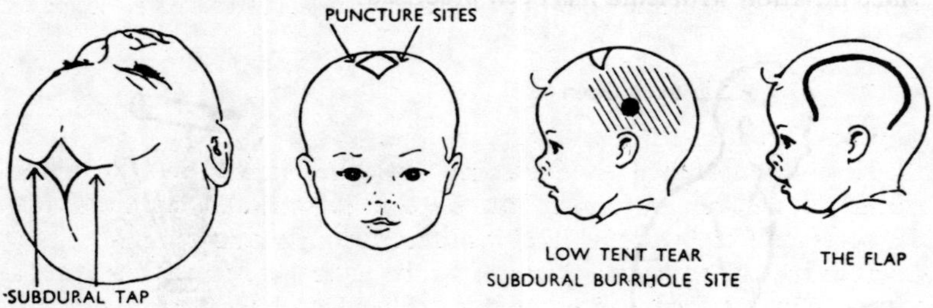

Armchair Corner

'Do noble deeds, not dream them. . .. '

Yet the philosopher may be excused a digression concerning the nature of the chronic subdural haematoma. Its site, distribution and nature are unlike those of the acute and subacute from which it might be expected to have arisen, whilst it never occurs after craniotomy when blood might reasonably be expected to have been left to encyst in the subdural space. Further, it commonly occurs under bone of consistency like that of early Paget's disease (the hyperaemic cheesy stage) and in association with haemorrhagic friable dura.

Is it an intradural haematoma, the result of splitting of the dura by a haemorrhage into it? Or is its development dependent upon an intact arachnoid without possibility of absorption of blood through the subarachnoid space?

But the armchair grows comfortable—back to work.

SUBDURAL HYGROMA

This is a wretched title which serves as cover for a hotch-potch of varied fluid collections in the subdural space. Some attempt at separation is needed.

(The subdural space is a most peculiar body plane in which many odd lesions occur. It is best compared with the pleural cavity. Thus the titles that follow.)

Hydrocranium

Compare this with pneumothorax.

At the time of injury the arachnoid may be torn so that cerebrospinal fluid escapes into the subdural space. Inspection holes may show a large, low pressure collection of fluid with a collapsed brain beneath it. Arterial hypotension from injury often co-exists at this early stage.

Tension Hydrocranium

Compare this with tension pneumothorax.

Here cerebrospinal fluid escapes through a flap valve tear in the arachnoid, and cannot return. The contused brain swells slightly, raising the pressure. Cerebrospinal fluid is pumped from a subarachnoid cistern (such as that of the sylvian fissure) by the pulsating brain. Thus arises a space-occupying and localized subdural collection under tension, presenting as would a haematoma.

Presentation is usually on the second to seventh day.

Treatment is by burrhole as for acute or subacute haematoma, and evacuation and drainage of the collection. Note that a collection of this sort may be adjacent to a subdural haematoma, and is quite common beneath an extradural haematoma as noted earlier.

The Posterior Fossa Collection

This is similar to the above condition. The arachnoid is torn and cerebrospinal fluid escapes over a cerebellar hemisphere. Cerebellar swelling from contusion causes tonsillar herniation and obstructs the downward escape of cerebrospinal fluid from the cisterna magna. The subdural collection increases and adds to the medullary coning.

Presentation is by development of symptoms and signs of posterior fossa pressure lesion on the second to seventh day.

Headache, stiff neck, unilateral or bilateral abducens palsy, papilloedema, and pyramidal and sometimes cerebellar signs may be seen.

Treatment is by burrhole in the posterior fossa, evacuating the subdural fluid (it gushes out), wide opening of the cisterna magna and reduction of tonsillar herniation. If cerebellar contusion is extensive, full posterior fossa decompression may be required.

Subdural Effusion

This is the only lesion of the group that even approximates the meaning of hygroma.

The lesion resembles the chronic subdural haematoma in site, high over the convexity, but consists of a collection of bright yellow high protein fluid.

Presentation is on the third to tenth day, with severe headache, often accurately localized, as the main symptom. Irritability, slight fever, irregularities of pulse and blood pressure, and minor neurological signs are common.

Treatment is by burrhole, evacuation, irrigation and drainage of the subdural space.

(Note that similar effusions may overlie meningitis, as pleural effusion overlies pneumonia, and may become infected as subdural abcess, comparable with empyema. But we digress.)

Chronic Subdural Hygroma

This is an alleged longstanding (months or years) collection of fluid in the subdural space, due to injury and responsible for headache and other sequelae.

Fully substantiated examples of this are excessively rare. Such collections are so common after air studies (a method frequently used for their 'detection') and as incidental findings at craniotomy, that their significance is at least questionable.

SPATAPOPLEXIE TRAUMATISCHE

Literally delayed apoplexy due to trauma, this condition is a stroke occurring one to three weeks after relatively minor injury. True examples exist where a haemorrhage occurs in an area known to have been injured, and remote from the usual site of strokes, in the absence of vascular disease.

The subject is of greater medico-legal than surgical importance.

RECOMMENDED FURTHER READING

Ingraham, F.S. and Matson, D.D. (1944). 'Subdural Haematoma in Infancy'. *J. Pediat.* **24**, 1

Jamieson, K.G. (1954). 'Delayed Traumatic Intracerebral Haemorrhage'. *Aust. N.Z. J. Surg.* **23**, 300

Trotter, W. (1914). 'Chronic Subdural Haemorrhage of Traumatic Origin and its Relation to Pachymeningitis Haemorrhagica Interna.' *Br. J. Surg.* 2, 271

12—Fits, Faints, Fugues, Fancies and Frenzies

Abnormality of brain function is to be expected after any injury, and unconsciousness and hemiplegia or other tangible disabilities are accepted without surprise by most observers. But should convulsive disorders or aberrations of behaviour appear, their significance is often ill understood.

Here we shall consider further the importance of fits, of other epileptic variants and of odd confusional states after injury.

Noisy restlessness and violent irritability, so often causes of annoyance to nursing staff and hospital administrators, must be considered in relation to their meaning in terms of the injury.

One of the greatest disservices that can be done to a patient is to administer sedatives and depress him without consideration of the reason for his behaviour.

'The patient's noisy—stop the row—
Shut him up—we don't care how!
Give him sedatives, tie him down!'
(Flat on back, to choke and drown).

So say the fools who can't assess
Or care for patients in distress.
Give sedatives? No—diagnose
Before the man turns up his toes.
If you insist he rest in peace,
R.I.P. may mean decease.

FITS

Epileptic fits may occur at any stage after injury; immediately, or after the passage of years. They are of importance for three reasons:

(*i*) their diagnostic significance;
(*ii*) their effect on general management; and
(*iii*) their therapeutic needs in their own right.

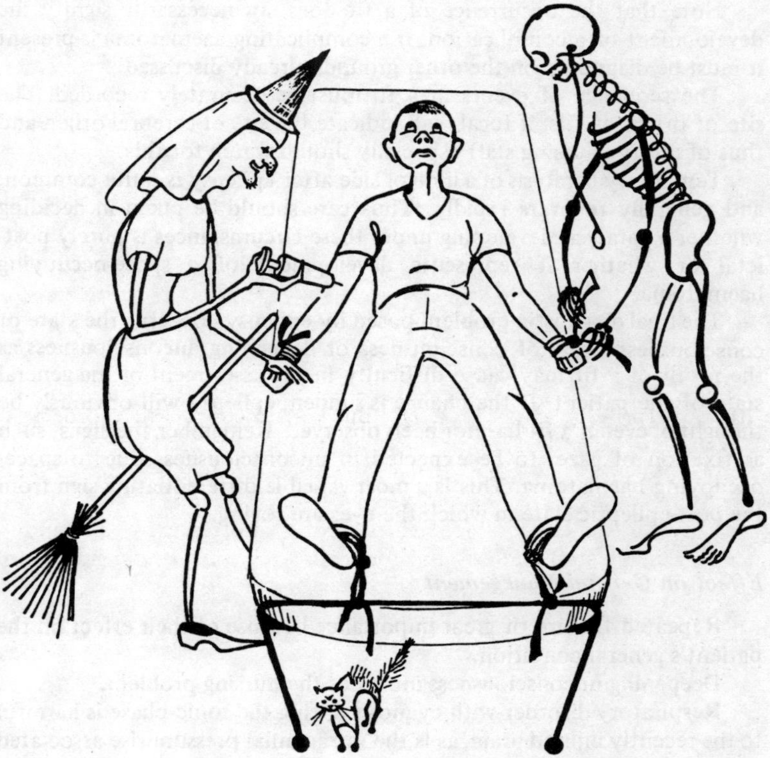

ABANDON HOPE ALL YE THAT ENTER HERE!

It must be stressed that epilepsy is not a disease, but a clinical symptom and sign of cerebral disorder which may have varied aetiology. Just as hemiplegia can occur from many causes, and may be of localizing value, so can epileptic fits.

Diagnostic Significance

The occurrence of an epileptic fit may be evidence of acute injury to, or irritation of, the brain. Cerebral contusion or laceration, intracerebral, subarachnoid or subdural haemorrhage may be the cause, but fits are very rare with extradural haemorrhage unless the brain has also been injured.

Note that the occurrence of a fit does not necessarily signify the development of a complication. If a complicating haematoma is present it must be diagnosed on the other grounds already discussed.

The sequence of events in a fit must be accurately recorded. The site of origin of fits, if focal, will indicate the site of cerebral origin and thus of injury. Nursing staff especially should watch for this.

Temporary paralysis of a limb or side after epilepsy is quite common, and generally recovers rapidly. Thus care should be taken in deciding whether a paralysis developing under these circumstances is purely post-ictal or whether it represents development of a space-occupying haematoma.

The final diagnostic problem posed by epilepsy concerns the state of consciousness. Loss of consciousness or deepening unconsciousness as the result of a fit may cause difficulty in the assessment of the general state of the patient. If the change is sudden, epilepsy will obviously be thought of even if a fit has not been observed. Remember the signs, such as fixation of gaze, to be expected in unconsciousness due to space-occupying haematoma. This is a most valuable differentiating sign from the post-epileptic state in which the eyes are roving.

Effect on General Management

Repeated fits are of great importance because of their effect on the patient's general condition.

Deepening unconsciousness increases the nursing problem.

Respiratory disorder with cyanosis during the tonic phase is harmful to the recently injured brain, as is the intracranial pressure rise associated with struggling.

Increased salivation during a fit increases the risk of aspiration pneumonia.

For all of these reasons fits must be stopped even at the risk of administering sedatives. This, however, by stopping the fits, is likely to improve the state of consciousness and make assessment of general progress simpler.

Therapy

In the acute phase, and for rapid control of fits, intramuscular barbiturates are the best drugs to use. Luminal 200 mg is a standard dosage. Should this fail, do not use Paraldehyde. Please note that this drug depresses consciousness much more (in effective dosage) and makes general assessment of the patient more difficult.

Dilantin 100 mg up to six times a day should be given early to ensure control. This dosage may be reduced gradually when control has been achieved.

In the acute phase, stop repeated fits at all costs if you can. Control is usually easy, but if intramuscular Luminal fails, give intravenous sodium amytal.

The management of post-traumatic epilepsy after the acute phase of head injury has passed is on routine anticonvulsant lines and need not be discussed here. Prescribe anticonvulsants, proscribe alcohol.

FAINTS, FUGUES AND FANCIES

Great care should be taken in the assessment of 'peculiar' states of consciousness, of apparently hysterical behaviour, and of hallucinations reported by the patient. Any of these states may be due to epilepsy, especially from temporal lobe lesions. Again this need not be discussed in full here, but the need for caution is stressed.

Especially be careful not to mistake complete aphasia, from injury to speech centres, for hysteria or unco-operative behaviour.

Post-traumatic amnesia of the graphic variety beloved of fiction authors is an extreme rarity.

FRENZIES

Confused noisy restlessness, violence and obscenity are quite common after injury, and should be assessed carefully. As stated earlier, increasing restlessness may be a sign of improvement in a patient emerging from concussion, or may be a sign of complication when consciousness deteriorates or remains unaltered.

Common causes of restlessness are increasing headache, forcible restraint of a confused patient, dehydration with acute thirst, and a full bladder or rectum.

Before you further restrain the patient or give sedatives, assess the cause. Craniotomy may be the correct treatment at times, administration of fluid or provision of a bedpan at others. Don't give sedatives blindly.

One of the greatest perils facing the patient who is noisy and restless is ill-considered sedation administered for the benefit of his attendants and neighbours in the ward. Such sedation may obscure complications until they are irreversible, and may precipitate the respiratory accidents which threaten the unconscious.

The role of the frontal lobe injury in producing this state has already been discussed. Give sedatives rationally, securing sleep for the patient at night, and mobilize him during the day. Tranquillizing drugs, such as Largactil, may be of more value than sedatives.

If you cannot control a violent patient and fear he may fall out of bed, nurse him on a mattress on the floor.

Headache

Severe headache requires relief which may sometimes be achieved by such simple measures as sitting the patients up, reducing noise and light, and administering aspirin or codeine compounds.

On other occasions more powerful drugs are required. Pethedine or opiates may have to be given but care should be taken not to depress respiration, and not to depress consciousness to a level at which assessment of progress of the patient would be difficult. Sometimes tranquillizing drugs provide good relief without undesirable side effects, while barbiturates may cause increasing confusion.

It has often been said that opiates are absolutely contra-indicated in the presence of head injury. Such an attitude is completely wrong, as is obvious especially in patients suffering multiple injury.

In each case assess the cause of headache or pain and apply the appropriate measures for relief. In each case select both drug and dosage with care, to avoid depressing respiration and disturbing consciousness unnecessarily.

RECOMMENDED FURTHER READING

Jennett, W.B. (1962). *Epilepsy after Blunt Head Injuries.* Heinemann London:

Walker, A.E. and Jablon, S. (1961). *Follow-up Study of Head Wounds in World War II,* pp. 35, 116. Veterans Administration Medical Monograph. Washington: U.S. Government Printing Office

– and Erculei, F. (1968). *Brain-injured Men.* Springfield, Ill.: Thomas

Part IV
Physiology and Nursing Care

To date our attention has been focused upon the isolated head, which must now be incorporated with the so-far decapitated body to allow us to view the patient as a whole.

Here we will consider the effects of head injury upon the body and the intracranial results of general complications. The intracranial events may be dramatic and demanding of our attention, but the more general matters of posture, of respiration and of hydration, to mention a few, may determine the outcome.

The person who does most for the patient with head injury is not the surgeon who performs the occasionally necessary operation, but the doctor and nurse who roll up their sleeves, position the patient correctly, secure him a free airway, and provide general care.

13—Respiration

'Noisy breathing is obstructed breathing'.

Anaesthetist's maxim

'If the face is blue, the brain is, too'.

Nursery rhyme

Bronchopneumonia has long been libelled as a common cause of death after head injury, and this has been advanced as a reason for care of respiration in the unconscious.

The reasoning represents:

(i) misuse of the term bronchopneumonia, as if patients with head injury were particularly liable to primary bacterial infection of their bronchi, and thus of the lung;

(ii) misunderstanding of the reason patients die when respiratory complications supervene; and

(iii) misrepresentation of the reason for care of the respiratory tract.

Certain it is that care of respiration is of vital importance in the management of head injury. Yet a measure of the lip-service paid to this principle is the dozen or so lines devoted to the subject by the author of each of two 400 page tomes on head injury.

ONE ACT PLAYS FOR TRAUMA SURGEONS

Play the First

'THE STUDENT NURSE IN SEARCH OF SENSE'

Setting: Any 'modern' hospital
Time: Regrettably, the present.

SCENE I

(The post-operative recovery room. Patients recovering from anaesthesia for various operations lie on trolleys or beds—according to the stage props available. Each lies strictly on his side, supported thus by his flexed lower limbs and by pillows. Each has his head turned slightly downwards so that saliva runs out on to a towel provided. Each has an airway. Many are attended by nurses holding the paralysed jaw forward. Suction apparatus is in evidence and in use; the atmosphere is one of efficiency and of hopeful expectancy.)

Enter student nurse (S.N.) who talks with recovery room supervisor (R.R.S.) and anaesthetist (A.).

S.N. Why are the patients on their sides?

R.R.S. Because they are unconscious. Gravity may kill the unconscious patient who lies on his back.

S.N. How come?

R.R.S. There are two reasons—respiratory obstruction and aspiration pneumonia.

S.N. Please explain.

R.R.S. Many muscles are flaccid as the result of anaesthetic unconsciousness. If the patient were on his back his cheeks, if he is edentulous, his soft palate and tongue, and his jaw, would fall back to obstruct the breathing. That is the reason for the airway and nurse who holds the jaw forward to keep the tongue forward.

S.N. What about the aspiration pneumonia?

R.R.S. The larynx is also paralysed and the patient cannot cough to protect his lungs from saliva or vomitus that might run under gravity down the pharynx and trachea. That is why the mouth is turned downward and the sucker is in use to remove secretions.

S.N. Why are these things important?

R.R.S. Both obstruction and pneumonia can produce anoxia which may. . . .

A. (interrupting) Sister, that patient's breathing is noisy and laboured—it is obviously obstructed—come and we will correct it. (They go to the patient and the doctor attends to the patient's needs, assisted by nursing staff.)

S.N. The patient appeared blue—don't you give oxygen for that?

A. No, you correct the cause of cyanosis by ensuring a free airway. You see, he is already pink, as soon as his breathing is quiet and easy.

Rose-coloured Curtain

(Appropriate to the pink patient and the general mood).

RESPIRATION

SCENE II

(The acute surgical wards. Consultant and resident staff are grouped about a bed occupied by a patient with bandaged belly and various tubes in sundry orifices. The patient is mildly cyanosed with rapid respirations and pulse rate. A doctor auscultates the chest while consultant, physiotherapist and sister encourage the patient to cough.)

Enter student nurse (S.N.) who talks with consultant (C.) and physiotherapist (P.).

S.N. What is wrong with this patient?

C. He has aspiration peneumonia. We are trying to clear his lungs by making him cough.

S.N. What else can be done?

C. If this fails we will use a bronchoscope to suck out the lungs, for this condition is serious and requires urgent attention.

S.N. What can be done to prevent it?

P. We turn the patient from side to side to allow drainage of the lungs, and thump his chest to dislodge plugs of mucus and encourage expectoration.

S.N. If it is pneumonia, don't you give antibiotics?

C. No, the problem is a purely mechanical one; once we clear the lungs, infection will not occur.

S.N. Do you usually succeed?

C. Of course, with proper care and enthusiasm.

White Curtain

(Appropriate to the gentle light of reason.)

SCENE III

(A general medical ward. The atmosphere is distinctly geriatric, for the physicians have already cured or prevented most medical diseases of youth. Several elderly, and some younger, patients lie flat on their backs, obviously unconscious, snoring violently or bubbling gently; a doctor sits at sister's desk, oblivious to the cacophony, earnestly writing.)

Enter student nurse who talks with doctor and sister.

S.N. Are these patients unconscious?

D. Of course.

S.N. But they are lying on their backs and I can hear mucus rattling in their tracheas!

S. That's the death rattle; it means they will soon die.

S.N. I should think they will. Can't something be done?

D. They suffer from strokes that we can't treat; I am busy with–(the name escapes the student nurse)–syndrome.

S.N. (aside) This must be a different sort of unconsciousness from the anaesthetic sort.

Blue Curtain

(Appropriate to the patient's colour and to the mood.)

SCENE IV

(Another surgical ward. A patient unconscious from head injury lies half on his back, half on his side, snoring violently. He is attended by a frightened junior nurse who is unable to improve the airway. Doctor again sits at the desk.)

Enter Student Nurse who talks with Junior Nurse (J.N.).

S.N. Why isn't the patient on his side, since he is unconscious?

J.N. Oh, but he is!

S.N. But he can't be far enough on his side because his breathing is rapid and noisy, and the anaesthetist says that means obstruction.

J.N. But this breathing is stertorous, and our books say that means cerebral compression.

S.N. What does stertorous mean?

J.N. I think it means noisy and laboured.

S.N. It sounds like snoring to me, and people only snore when they're on their backs.

J.N. Oh, but this is different—our books say so.

S.N. Can't Doctor do anything?

J.N. No, he says operation wouldn't help.

Grey Curtain

(Appropriate to ignorance and the mists of uncertainty.)

SCENE V

(The Casualty Department. An accident victim is carried in. Blood trickles from a forehead wound and he is clearly unconscious. He lies flat on his back, his respiration is rapid and laboured, and with each breath vomitus bubbles from his lips. What can be seen of his face is blue and congested.)

The conversation piece is limited to bubbling and gasping noises. Exit student nurse, confused and lost for words.

Sickly Green Curtain

SCENE VI

(The hospital mortuary. Sundry mortal remains with the usual props.)

Enter student nurse who talks with not-so-morbid anatomist (N-S-M. A.).

N-S-M. A. Hullo, Nurse. Come and see what killed this head injury.

S.N. But that isn't his brain, it's his lungs.

N-S-M. A. Yes, and see how wet they are. Silted up with saliva and mucus and so on.

S.N. Is that bronchopneumonia?

N-S-M. A. No, it is hypostatic and inhalation pneumonia from the effect of gravity and a paralysed larynx in the unconscious.

S.N. Then we should be able to prevent it.

N-S-M. A. Yes, but you sometimes fail and sometimes even help it. That one over there died of egg-flip in the bronchi.

S.N. Then the brain is all right and the lungs kill the patient?

N-S-M. A. Not quite, for the obstruction to breathing caused by a blocked airway or by fluid in the lungs affects the brain.

S.N. Can you show me how?

N-S-M. A. Come and look at this one. He died of suffocation, obstruction of his airway.

S.N. But now you're showing me the brain, not the lungs.

N-S-M. A. Of course; see how swollen it is? And when I cut it, what do you see?

S.N. Little haemorrhages all through it. Is that what respiratory obstruction does to the brain?

N-S-M. A. You've got the picture.

Black and Final Curtain

Play the Second

'FREE AIR OR GO FLAT'

Cast: Gas station attendant – anaesthetist (A.)
Chief mechanic – surgeon (S.)
Assistant mechanic (R.M.O.)

Setting: Again the hospital

Time: Still the present.

SCENE I

(The operating theatre. A patient with cerebral tumour lies on the table, osteoplastic flap cut and dura open. The brain bulges slightly, the surface veins are dilated and congested.)

RESPIRATION

A. That brain looks rather tight; I'll check the respiration and my connections again.

S. Thank you, but I think this is just due to tumour.

A. Yes, everything is all right here.

R.M.O. Can the anaesthetist cause high pressure?

S. Not this one. We choose our anaesthetists carefully because they don't have accidents. But if an endotracheal tube is kinked, the vessels become engorged, and brain herniates and ruptures. It is a most dramatic and frightening event which our anaesthetist spares us.

R.M.O. What is the mechanism?

S. The most powerful of all cerebral vasodilators is carbon dioxide. If you lumbar puncture a patient and let him rebreathe into a bag, his lumbar pressure will rise rapidly. Carbon dioxide retention is the most potent cause of cerebral venous congestion and high intracranial pressure. The anaesthetist knows this and double checks, leaving nothing to chance.

Sterile Curtain

SCENE II

(The tea room, between operations. The scene is familiar enough to require no stage directions.)

R.M.O. I thought our care of the respiratory tract was designed to prevent bronchopneumonia as a complication of head injury. Now I see that we are preventing raised intracranial pressure.

S. But that is only part of the story. If you have a clear concept of the state of the brain after injury–bruised and torn–what do you think will happen if venous congestion is produced by inadequate care of respiration?

R.M.O. The injured brain will become oedematous and bleed. Even subdural and intracerebral haematomas may be produced.

S. Now do you see that care of respiration is the most important and direct way we have of arresting and preventing haemorrhage from the injured brain?

A. Not to mention anoxia!

S. Yes, prolonged anoxia will certainly increase the brain damage and the final neurological deficit.

Curtain–of Cigarette Smoke

SCENE III

(The neurosurgeon's home at dead of night. The telephone rings.)

S. Hullo.

. . . .

S. But he was almost talking earlier, and now you say he's unconscious, with only sluggish response to painful stimuli.

. . . .

S. I don't think he is likely to have an extradural from what I remember of his injury, but I'll come and see.

. . . .

S. Is his respiration quite all right, not noisy and obstructed?

. . . .

S. That doesn't sound at all adequate. I'll be with you soon.

(Dresses and exits)

Considerable time lapse.

Surgeon re-enters.

Wife. Did you have to operate?

S. No, just my usual night call–a head injury that had gone off because his breathing was obstructed. He's obeying commands again now. Put him on his side, suck him out properly, see that he responds and go home as usual.

Dawn-coloured Curtain

Play the Third

'AS WE'D LIKE IT'

Setting: Lecture room and ward.

Time: As often as possible.

(The scene is formal or informal, as opportunity presents. The nursing staff are instructed in the care of the unconscious.)

Enter the lecturer or demonstrator, who speaks much as follows:

'Care of respiration is of vital importance in head injury management. The person who does most for the patient is not the surgeon who performs the occasionally necessary operation, but the doctor or nurse who rolls up his sleeves, positions the patient correctly, secures him a free airway and provides general care.

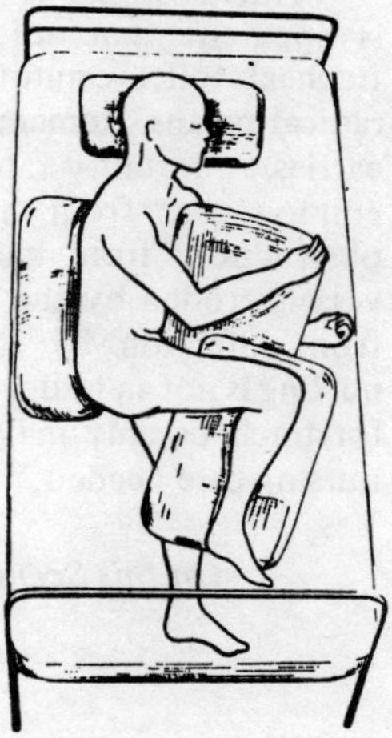

'*Position.* Place the patient on his side with hips and knees flexed, a pillow between the thighs and another behind the back to stabilize him. Both arms should be in front of the patient. If you put one under him (as in Sim's position used for short-term unconsciousness) he will tend to roll onto his face and his body-weight might then impede respiration. Turn the face mouth-downward to drain saliva. Change the patient on to alternate sides at least four-hourly to promote postural drainage of the lungs and to relieve pressure areas.

'*Airway.* Ensure quiet unobstructed breathing. An oral, or sometimes a nasopharyngeal, airway will often assist. Clear the airway often; it tends to become occluded with dried secretions.

'*Suck out* accumulating nasal secretions, saliva, vomitus (the large alcoholic meal that precipitated the accident), blood and cerebrospinal fluid before they are aspirated. Suck out through the nostrils for best access to the pharynx, and empty the pool in the dependent cheek.

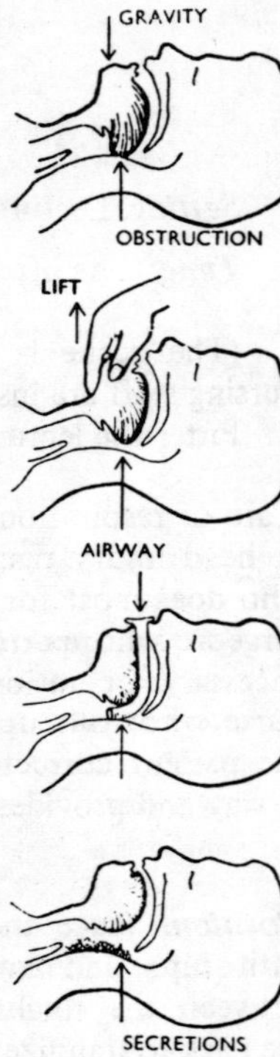

'*Empty* the full stomach and don't fill it again to regurgitate in the acute phase.

'*Reduce secretions;* control epilepsy, don't use irritating indwelling duodenal tubes for feeding or hydration until a cough reflex is re-established.

'*Laryngoscope* and suck out the trachea when necessary, bronchoscope if indicated.

'*Tracheostomy* is warranted as soon as it is apparent that an adequate airway and tracheal toilet cannot be provided by less radical means. Remember that tracheostomy carries a mortality rate in its own right from emphysema, from tracheal crusting and obstruction, from haemorrhage from those vessels eroded by the tube on occasion, and from infection by the sucker. Inadequate nursing is not an indication for tracheostomy, for tracheostomy may then but increase the nursing care needed.'

On this Scene–No Curtain

Problem Corner

Pulmonary Oedema

Neurogenic pulmonary oedema is an occasional acute complication of head injury, recognized by the expectoration or aspiration of stringy viscid mucus followed by the welling out of pink froth from the lungs.

The treatment of this condition is to intubate the patient's trachea with a cuffed tube and provide positive pressure respiration. A small rise in intra-alveolar pressure is sufficient to prevent the escape of fluid from the lung capillaries, and indeed to promote re-absorption of fluid that has already escaped.

Tracheostomy or other endeavours to suck out the patient are usually unavailing; blow the fluid back in!

Depressed Respiration

When respiration is depressed, carbon dioxide retention readily occurs with all its potential risks. Therefore give no respiratory depressant drugs; avoid opiates and over-sedation. If depression is spontaneous or established, endeavour to stimulate respiration. The half-hourly disturbance of the patient during observation serves a therapeutic as well as a diagnostic purpose for this reason. An endotracheal tube or a tracheostomy may be useful, since they reduce the dead-space and improve the efficiency of respiration.

Maintaining an Airway

When difficulty is experienced in maintaining a free airway by posture and a pharyngeal airway, endotracheal intubation (per-oral at first, converted to per-nasal) using a Portex tube is desirable. Such a tube not only secures an airway but aids bronchotracheal toilet with suction catheters using strict aseptic techniques.

Portex tubes may be left down for 24–48 hours in adults or for much longer in infants without laryngeal damage – but red rubber ones may not. Such management should precede tracheostomy except in dire emergency, and tracheostomy is then possible as an elective procedure for longer term cases under ideal conditions with an endotracheal tube in place for the operation.

It must be remembered that an artificial airway must be looked after just as much as a natural one. It is subject to displacement upwards or downwards into a bronchus, and to obstruction by kinking or accumulation within it of inspissated secretions. Ability to pass a suction catheter through it is not guarantee of patency of a sufficient lumen for breathing – if in doubt, change the tube.

Humidification of inspired air by an appropriate nebulizer is essential when the normal mechanisms of humidification in the upper respiratory tract have been bypassed. Dehydration of the patient predisposes to thick adherent secretions; adequate hydration is important to successful bronchotracheal toilet. Mucolytics should be avoided since their pH is damaging to function of cilia.

Assisted Respiration

Tachypnoea may or may not mean hyper-ventilation – in some cases respiration is so shallow that tidal air only is exchanged. On other occasions in severe injury true hyper-ventilation may occur with severe respiratory alkalosis. In either circumstance artificial ventilation may be of benefit in maintaining normal blood gases.

14—Intracranial Pressure and Posture

Next time you see a child swinging upside-down on the 'monkey-bars', look at its face. There you will see the venous congestion that occurs when the head is lowered beneath the level of the heart. Reflect that when the pathologist wishes to congest a vein to obtain blood, he hangs the limb below the level of the heart and obstructs the venous return.

If you wish to make the bruised and torn brain bleed, raise the foot of the bed!

If you wish to arrest or prevent haemorrhage, sit the patient up as soon as it is safe to do so, nurse him flat until then. You cannot sit him up until his cough reflex and consciousness return.

The only excuses for putting the foot of the bed on blocks are: (*i*) the presence of shock, which is rare in head injury unless blood loss from scalp has been excessive, or there are associated injuries; and (*ii*) vomiting, to prevent inhalation of vomitus during the act.

If the patient has associated lower limb fractures requiring traction against body weight, make sure that his head is raised.

The efficacy of venous return from the head is one of the important factors in determining the intracranial pressure.

Raised Intracranial Pressure

Soon after injury, the intracranial pressure is often raised. That is, an increased intracraniospinal content stretches the elastic dural container where it can yield at cranial foraminae and within the spinal canal. Thus the occurrence of headache.

The increased intracranial content may be haematoma, may be subarachnoid blood (with resultant excessive cerebrospinal fluid secretion), may be oedema and brain swelling, and may be venous congestion.

As the pressure rises, the intracranial circulation is embarrassed by pressure collapse of those vessels with the lowest intraluminal pressure; the terminal veins as they enter the great dura-lined and incompressible venous sinuses. The effect of terminal vein compression is to produce vascular congestion in the brain and further raise the pressure, a vicious circle mechanism.

Embarrass the venous return and you may initiate this disastrous sequence.

Do not obstruct the jugulars; ensure natural head position. Especially when the patient is on his side a low pillow may be necessary. The days of 'nurse flat, no pillow' went out with the six weeks darkened room treatment of concussion. Watch that tracheotomy tapes are not tied too tightly.

The Relation of Pressure and Posture

In the normal lateral position used for lumbar puncture, the intracranial pressure equals that found at lumbar puncture, 50–150 mm of cerebrospinal fluid. When the patient sits up, the column of fluid in a spinal manometer stands to the level of the foramen magnum. Above that, the pressure is subatmospheric. Drill a hole in the head of a sitting patient, and air runs in. Thus by merely sitting the patient up, the intracranial pressure can be lowered from the normal recumbent level of 50–150 mm of fluid to subatmospheric. This is the most effective and physiological method available for lowering the intracranial pressure! As soon as the patient's cough reflex is safe, sit him up if you want his pressure lowered!

Obstruct the internal jugular veins during lumbar puncture, as in Queckenstedt's test, or have the patient obstruct the venous return by the Valsalva manoeuvre, and you will see the immediate effect of cerebrospinal venous congestion on intracranial pressure. Picture what happens within the head of a restrained and struggling patient! Think again of the effects of respiratory embarrassment!

Classically, the headache of raised intracranial pressure is worst in the early morning when the patient wakens from the recumbency and respiratory depression of sleep, and passes off when he gets up, breathes up and moves about.

What Not to do to Patients

Consider the case of a man suffering an undiagnosed cerebral tumour, producing symptoms of headache and a limp, but allowing him to go about his usual daily routine until he consults a doctor.

He is then likely to be put to bed in a hospital so that gravity no longer aids his venous return, and given sedatives to depress him and his respiration to ensure a night's sleep. Opiates or pethedine may be administered to reduce his discomfort during an angiogram or air study, thus increasing the depression and killing him with kindness. An unnecessary anaesthetic may increase the depression, while a lumbar puncture may further disturb his intracranial hydrodynamics.

Within hours or days his intracranial pressure may reach the critical level at which the venous return is embarrassed so that cerebral venous congestion supervenes. Thus unconsciousness and a surgical emergency may be precipitated not by further growth of the tumour, but by meddlesome interference with those physiological mechanisms that allow it to be accommodated within the skull.

The patient with a chronic subdural haematoma often exhibits fluctuation in consciousness. On one day he is awakened, washed, sat up, stimulated to eat breakfast, and got out of bed. He has a wakeful day. On another day falsely placed sympathy or overwork on the part of his attendants dictates that he is allowed to lie unstimulated. That is a day of stupor.

Do not remove gravity from the patient's aid unnecessarily.

Do not permit respiratory depression.

Do not depress respiration with opiates, sedatives or needless anaesthetics.

Think of what you are doing!

15—Shock and Associated Injuries

Many patients who suffer head injuries sustain other injuries. The problems that arise are:

(1) Resuscitation and assessment of the injured patient as a whole.
(2) Allocation of priorities in treatment.

The doctor was waiting in Cas. as they brought
The injured man in through the door.
'He's suffering blood loss, and collapse', he thought,
'And his breathing I just can't ignore'.
The patient was struggling and gasping for breath,
The whole of his chest wall was flapping;
Respiratory paradox had him near death—
Quite useless to think of just strapping.
An endotracheal cuffed tube was soon passed,
Respiratory control was full;
They blew up his lungs with firm pressure; at last
His breathing was not push and pull.
A drip was produced, quickly placed in a vein,
And albumen given post haste;
His blood was cross-matched, and while this was in train
More fluid—there's no time to waste.
His B.P. came up and his pulse rate soon slowed;
Fresh bleeding occurred from an arm;
Firm pressure arrested it—had it still flowed
A forceps would soon stop the harm.
They splinted his fractures in manner first-aid
To lessen the trauma and pain,
Examined his belly, and thorough search made
For rupture of viscus—in vain.
The next was his head, with a bruise on the brow,
Beneath it the bone was depressed;
This wasn't the cause of the shock, so till now

Could wait till the rest was assessed.
So that is the order when multiple blows
Rain down on the poor human frame;
The breathing, blood volume, then head down to toes
According to each member's claim.

Shock

'Surgical shock', nowadays an unfashionable term, does not occur in head injury unless it is overwhelmingly severe or there is much external blood loss. Since the volume of tissue injured is small, circulating volume is not much reduced except in the large subgaleal haematoma of infancy.

If the patient is shocked, seek another injury–limbs, pelvis, abdomen or thorax–which may be more urgent.

Resuscitate before you operate unless the head injury is clearly the most urgent lesion. Then resuscitate while you operate.

Respiratory Distress

Think of the chest!

Many thoracic injuries are missed because there is little external bruising through the patient's clothing. Severe pulmonary injury and pneumo- or haemothorax can occur without fracture, because the thoracic cage is so elastic that it is poor protection for the lungs.

Many a patient with bruise on head and crushed chest is suspected of intracranial haemorrhage when he lapses into unconsciousness, only to waken dramatically when his pneumothorax is aspirated!

Remember the signs of hypercapnia–raised blood pressure and tachycardia, with or without sweating. Cyanosis from anoxia may be completely absent. Be sure that the trachea and bronchi are not full of blood or vomitus in the comatose patient. If you assist respiration and remove excess carbon dioxide, the blood pressure may fall dramatically when this stimulus disappears. Be ready to support the circulation.

Relieve respiratory distress before you operate, and be certain the airway if free throughout the operation.

Abdominal Injuries

Abdominal injuries frequently co-exist with head injury, especially after traffic accidents. Look for the superficial bruising, the local tenderness, the signs of free fluid or blood, and the rigidity.

In the drowsy or unconscious patient, no symptoms may be available. In the presence of rigidity from brain injury, it may be very difficult to determine the presence of an intra-abdominal lesion. The only clue may be the expiratory grunting associated with diaphragmatic irritation, which is quite different from the respiration of airway obstruction or brainstem dysfunction.

Facial Injuries

Facial injuries are often associated with cranial ones; don't miss the zygoma, the nose, the mandible and the centre-block face!

Cervical Spine

Most injuries to the head involve energy expended on the cervical spine. Look for fracture or fracture dislocation.

Limb Injuries

Fat embolism may occur, and produces fever, tachycardia, deterioration of consciousness and sometimes death, with incidence usually at about 24–48 hours. Petechial haemorrhages, found especially in the lower conjunctival sac and on the anterior axillary wall, aid differential diagnosis.

Fitness for Anaesthesia

How soon may a patient with head injury be anaesthetized, perhaps to treat a fractured limb? The answer depends upon the relative urgency of the operation to be conducted compared with the necessity for observation of the patient, assuming that the anaesthetic will be skilfully administered with neither anoxia nor hypercapnia.

Wait if you can until the head injury position is stable.

Watch all the more closely during anaesthesia.

RECOMMENDED FURTHER READING

Jamieson, K.G. and Tait, I.A. (1966). *'Traffic Injury in Brisbane. Report of a General Survey'. National Health and Medical Research Council Special Report Series,* No. 13, p.354. Canberra, Australia.

16—Routine Care of the Unconscious

The following reminders concerning general nursing care may be appropriate.

Hydration

A young man was hit on the head,
'He soon should be better', they said.
But they left out his drip,
He dried up like a chip.
And, 'ere they all knew it, was dead

Much has been written of dehydration therapy in head injury, as an endeavour to reduce oedema and intracranial pressure. This farce is seen at its best when rectal magnesium sulphate is given a patient receiving intravenous fluids. Dehydration may be reasonable in the first 24 hours, except in infants and the elderly, but after that the full daily physiological requirement of fluid must be given.

Hydrate, but don't overhydrate. Hypotonic and hyposmolar fluids should be avoided in parenteral therapy. An adequate electrolyte content should be assured by the balanced use of such solutions as Hartmann's in 5 per cent glucose, isosmotic glucose—saline, and stable plasma protein solution if cerebral oedema is to be prevented.

Intravenous fluids are the safest measure at first in the unconscious. The subcutaneous route carries great risk of staphylococcal infection in hospitals. Duodenal tube feeding carries the risk of regurgitation from the stomach and increase in salivation in the early phase. Change to oral fluids as soon as it is safe to do so.

Accurate input and output charts should be kept and will depend upon the ability to measure the urine of the unconscious.

Especially in warm weather, dehydration may be the cause of non-specific deterioration in the unconscious patient's condition; always consider the possibility. Thirst may be the cause of restlessness in the semiconscious.

Remember diabetes insipidus as a possible cause of dehydration.

Nutrition

A lassie was put on the table
Cut open by surgeon most able–
  Applause from the galleries.
  (But no salt or calories,
Forgotten, at last killed poor Mabel.)

Electrolyte imbalance readily occurs with parenteral feeding, especially with frontal lobe injury. Glucose and proteins can be administered.

Feeding via a stomach tube carries risks of bowel disturbance, especially of enteritis. Possibly vitamized meals are better than 'high protein fluids'.

Bladder

A man passed his water in bed
Till the skin on his back was quite red.
  A catheter passed
  Stopped his trouble at last
(He got pyelitis instead).

Collection of urine in the unconscious patient is desirable both to prevent bed-wetting (and thus frequent change) and to allow a fluid balance chart to be kept. Endeavours to catch the urine in a bottle may or may not be successful. External appliances, like a penile sheath, carry less risk of infection than catheterization, but urinary infection should be watched for and treated vigorously. Prolonged catheter drainage must be intermittent if a contracted bladder is to be avoided.

Calculus formation from urinary tract hypostasis is another risk in long-standing unconsciousness.

Bowels

A man with a large haematoma
Awoke after some weeks of coma;
  His bowels were impacted
  And when they first acted
The epic was worthy of Homer.

Simple care of the bowels, including use of suppositories, enemata and digital disimpaction, should be remembered.

Skin

A lad lay unconscious and spurned–
Not powdered, not rubbed and not turned;
  His bedding was wet–
  And what did he get?
The bedsores his nursing had earned.

Attention to pressure areas is very important, together with avoidance of all the factors that produce bedsores.

Joints and Muscles

A girl with a blow on the pate
Lay inert until much too late.
  Her hip joints were flexed
  And adducted–vexed,
The physios. can't get her straight!

Early full range passive movement of all limbs is essential to prevent contractures. Regular periods of nursing face down (when possible) will reduce the tendency to hip joint flexion.

Myositis ossificans occasionally occurs.

General Toilet

There was a young maiden, quite fair
Till doctors neglected her care–
  The corneas broke
  And crusting did choke
Her mouth and her teeth and her hair.

Eye toilet to prevent exposure keratitis, mouth toilet to clean away inspissated saliva and mucus and prevent respiratory tract infection, and general nursing care, are essential as well as humane.

Hope

A man with a broken right femur
Was strung up for months like a lemur.
He read comic papers,
Indulged in odd capers,
Behaved like a regular screamer.
The nurse in the ward was unworried–
The time lapse left her quite unflurried;
'For femurs to knit
It takes time, and it
Is something that just can't be hurried'.
But men who from head blows are reeling
May lie but a few days unfeeling
When every young nurse
Will look for the hearse–
Yet brains too take some time in healing!

RECOMMENDED FURTHER READING

Hooper, R.S. (1964). *Neurosurgical Nursing,* pp. 126, 127. Springfield, Ill.: Thomas

Lewin, W. (1966). *The Management of Head Injuries.* London: Baillière, Tindall & Cassell

McLaurin, R.L. (1966). 'Some Metabolic Aspects of Head Injury'. *Head Injury Conference Proceedings,* Ed. by W.F. Caveness and A.E. Walker. Philadelphia: Lippincott; London: Pitman

King, L.R., Elam, E.G. and Budde, R.B. (1960). 'Metabolic Response to Craniocerebral Trauma'. *Surgery Gynec. Obstet.* **110**, 282

Part V
Summary—Management of your Patient

For ease of discussion the many different facets of head injury have been dissected and dealt with separately in the main text.

Here our purpose is to assemble all those factors into a brief routine of appraisal and management of your particular patient, step by step from the injury.

Initial Diagnosis

Obtain a history of the injury and of the patient's state since injury, examine the head, and perform simple neurological examination.

Diagnose the degree and type of injury to scalp, skull and brain.

Predict the nature and site of possible complications in relation to the known mechanism of the injury.

Establish a Baseline

Record the state of the patient since injury, assess the state of consciousness and note pulse rate, blood pressure, respiration and temperature.

Establish thus a baseline from which subsequent changes can be evaluated.

Consider whether a complication had already become established before the patient was first seen.

Recognize the nature of concussion.

Institute Nursing Care

Correct position of nursing,
Prevention of respiratory obstruction,
Prevention of aspiration pneumonia,
Attention to hydration will allow your patient to survive.

Primary Indications for Operation

Scalp suture and elevation of fractures, with meticulous attention to detail, should be done as soon as resuscitation is completed and observation established.

Detection of Complications

Continued observation of the patient is the basis of detection of complications. Accurate assessment of the state of consciousness is the most important single feature.

Any evidence of deterioration at an interval after injury, whether in state of consciousness, neurological signs, size and reaction of pupils, pulse rate, blood pressure, respiration or temperature, is a sign that a complication is present.

Critical assessment of minimal signs of complication is the only means of early diagnosis and treatment while prognosis is good. Delay increases difficulty and invites disaster.

Differential Diagnosis of Complications

In some cases the type of deterioration suffered by the patient is so specific as to indicate the presence of a haematoma with certainty. The classical course of an extradural haematoma is an example. In other cases, the course of the patient shows no such specific features but the lesion may be essentially the same.

Consider the following checking list.

Respiration

Is respiration quiet, of normal rate, and not impeded?

Is the patient's colour good?

Is lung aeration good?

Otherwise, correct position of nursing and of jaw and tongue, provide an airway, aspirate the nasopharynx and pharynx, perform tracheal toilet by laryngoscopy or bronchoscopy, consider tracheostomy.

If respiration is rapid without local difficulty, measure the rectal temperature.

Remember the possibility of associated injury to the chest, especially in traffic accidents.

SUMMARY – MANAGEMENT OF YOUR PATIENT

Circulation

Is the circulation stable and adequate?

Are there signs of surgical shock or haemorrhage?

Again consider the possibility of associated injuries, especially to thorax and abdomen, with internal haemorrhage.

Is hydration adequate?

Temperature

Is the rectal temperature elevated?

Consider the possibilities:

(*i*) Neurogenic hyperthermia; the unmistakable clinical pciture.

(*ii*) Meningitis; is the injury compound (externally or into accessory nasal sinuses or ear)? Are there symptoms and signs of meningitis– headache, photophobia, stiff neck? Lumbar puncture if in doubt.

(*iii*) Infection elsewhere, especially lungs, or urinary tract after catheterization.

(*iv*) Dehydration.

Other Injuries

Associated injuries are common.

Look for them to account for unexplained respiratory difficulty or shock, and remember fat embolism.

Epilepsy

Has the patient suffered a fit?

Are there signs to suggest this, especially if deterioration in state of consciousness has been sudden?

Remember post-epileptic paralysis.

Are the eyes roving?

Haematoma

Remember that there may be no localizing signs, no pupil changes, no bradycardia or hypertension, no change in respiratory rhythm, no lucid interval.

Do not await the full classical picture, for the results are then classical and excessively bad.

If you cannot account for deterioration in any other way, you must operate.

Where to Seek Haematomas

If there are good localizing signs, use them, but otherwise, and in any case, explore as follows:

(1) At the site of the scalp bruise or the associated fracture line, seeking an extradural haematoma.

(2) Low in the temporal fossa on each side, seeking a subdural haematoma.

If you find a haematoma, follow it in the direction of increasing depth and expose it fully.

Remember to attend to respiration, prepare for blood loss, shave the scalp adequately, mark the incision before draping while you are still orientated, and illuminate properly.

Post-operative Course

If the patient deteriorates after operation, think of:

(*i*) re-accumulation of the primary haematoma;

(*ii*) post-operative extradural or subdural haemorrhage;

(*iii*) development of a new haematoma elsewhere; and

(*iv*) infection.

These diagnoses may be established on the general principles enumerated. If in doubt, reopen the wound.

Appendix 1

Special Investigations and Surgical Techniques

SPECIAL INVESTIGATIONS

Lumbar puncture	Air encephalography
Plain x-ray	Electro-encephalography
Angiography	Echo-encephalography
Ventriculography	Isotope studies

Lumbar Puncture

Mention of lumbar puncture has been almost absent from the text. The reason for this is that it is almost useless in the investigation and management of head injury, while contra-indications to its use are often present.

Indications

Detection of abnormal contents in the cerebrospinal fluid. – (*i*) *Pus.* The possibility of meningitis is a strong indication for lumbar puncture. If you seriously suspect it, it must be diagnosed or excluded.

(*ii*) *Blood.* Knowledge that there is blood in the cerebrospinal fluid is rarely of assistance. If the patient has localizing signs when first seen and doubt exists as to whether this is due to an extradural haematoma or a cerebral laceration, lumbar puncture might seem indicated. But the presence of blood in the fluid does not exclude either an extradural or a subdural haemorrhage, while the presence of space-occupying haematoma, especially in the posterior fossa with neck stiffness, makes lumbar puncture perilous. On rare occasions when post-traumatic subarachnoid haemorrhage is suspected, proof of the diagnosis may warrant puncture.

(*iii*) *Xanthochromia.* The presence of altered blood pigment at a considerable interval after minor trauma is a valuable sign of chronic subdural haematoma. Lumbar puncture at this relatively remote stage is a useful procedure.

Measurement of pressure. – When doubt exists in a patient who is otherwise healthy as to whether headache is due to raised pressure or to 'post-concussional syndrome' or 'post-traumatic neurosis', measurement of lumbar pressure may give a useful lead to diagnosis.

Contra-indications

Raised intracranial pressure. – It has already been seen that space-occupying haematomata commonly cause distortion of the brain and its herniation at either the tentorial orifice or the foramen magnum. Lumbar puncture under these circumstances may increase the degree of 'coning' and thus the brainstem dysfunction present.

When clinical signs of space-occupying lesion exist, lumbar puncture is to be avoided.

Before proceeding to lumbar puncture, examine the fundi. Papilloedema is a definite contra-indication to lumbar puncture on almost all occasions; certainly if surgical aid is not available immediately if the puncture causes deterioration.

Note that 'coning' is not necessarily immediately apparent; it may simply be accelerated so that death occurs at an interval.

Queckenstedt's test. – This test, performed by compression of the internal jugular veins during lumbar puncture, is a test of patency of the spinal theca. It thus has no place in the investigation of intracranial conditions except occasionally, and not very reliably, as a test for sinus thrombosis. It is *not* a routine part of lumbar puncture.

The only obstruction likely to be found by Queckenstedt's test in a case of intracranial lesion is a tentorial or medullary hernia, and he who performs Queckenstedt's test under these circumstances is attempting deliberately to strangulate such a hernia.

There is no defence for the negligence of a doctor who performs Queckenstedt's test when the pressure is high.

The pressure below a spinal block is always low or normal.

Plain X-ray

X-ray of the skull is desirable in all severe cases of head injury, for clinical as well as medico-legal purposes.

The support obtained for clinical diagnosis of fracture, or the detection of fracture in the absence of clinical signs, may give valuable information regarding the mechanism and site of trauma.

Radiographs of depressed fracture will indicate whether the inner table is splintered and thus the likelihood of dural and cerebral tearing, and the degree of penetration into the brain, as well as what structures such as venous sinuses may be involved.

Shift of the pineal (when visible) from the midline or asymmetry of the choroid plexuses (when calcified) may indicate the presence of a haematoma.

Presence of air within the skull – in the ventricles, or in the chiasmatic area in the brow-up lateral projection – indicates injury of the cribriform plate or accessory nasal sinuses and the risk of infection.

Follow-up x-rays, when indicated, may reveal such complications as osteomyelitis, erosion of fissure fractures in children, or ossification of a cephalhaematoma.

BUT Don't send patients to x-ray until their respiration is secure.
Don't send ill patients to x-ray unattended.
Don't waste time with x-rays when the patient will be safe only in the operating theatre.

Angiography

Carotid, and vertebral, angiography is a useful means of detection of space-occupying haematomata and determination of their site. However, it is by no means necessary and only occasionally used in very urgent cases even when it is available, which it is only in major centres. Interpretation of the films may require some little experience, and good quality films are a prerequisite to proper interpretation.

In less urgent cases when the pattern of complication evolves on a slower time base, angiography is extremely valuable for detecting intracranial haematomas and for differentiation of their type and site. Displacement of cerebral vessels together with surface avascular areas are the findings of importance, while medial displacement of a middle meningeal artery (and sometimes escape of dye from it) may aid diagnosis of extradural haemorrhage.

Especially when haematomas are in atypical sites, angiographic evidence may be most helpful in planning surgery, while assessment of post-operative problems is also more readily made when angiography is available.

Ventriculography

Air ventriculography is a more readily available special radiological technique, which may be useful both in infants and in older patients when clinical means of localization fail and routine exploratory surgery fails to disclose a haematoma.

Infants. – Pass a needle through the lateral angle of the anterior fontanelle, at right angles to scalp in all planes, to a depth, varying with age, of about 3 cm until cerebrospinal fluid is obtained. Cautiously withdraw fluid and replace with air.

Older children and adults. – Drill a burrhole at a point 11 cm above the external occipital protuberance and 3 cm lateral to the midline. Open the dura and into the brain pass a long blunt needle, aimed at the nasion, to a depth of 5–7 cm. When fluid is obtained, again withdraw some and replace with air, a few ml at a time.

Position the Head Carefully

Views. – Antero-posterior, brow up; lateral, brow up; postero-anterior, brow down; lateral brow down, and ordinary laterals will show any gross asymmetry of the ventricles and indicate the site of a haematoma. Failure of air to pass down the aqueduct into the fourth ventricle may indicate a posterior fossa lesion, as will displacement of the fourth ventricle.

Air Encephalography

Filling of the ventricles by injection of air through a lumbar puncture needle is a much less useful and more dangerous technique in the recent head injury. It combines the dangers of lumbar puncture with the even greater risks of large-scale withdrawal of fluid. Its use is to be discouraged, except in most dire necessity, even when ventriculography cannot be performed. There is, of course, no place for any of these studies unless it is intended and possible to proceed forthwith to any surgery indicated.

Electro-encephalography

This is mentioned chiefly to indicate awareness of its existence. We have not used it in investigation of the recently injured patient, though it commonly aids us in the management of post-traumatic epilepsy.

Echo-encephalography

Detection of midline shift, or of a cerebral surface echo away from the skull, by echo-encephalography may be most helpful, especially in doubtful cases and in children. However the technique, like most others, requires equipment, care, and experience in its use if valid results are to be obtained. As with other special investigations its use does not replace clinical assessment and must not be allowed to delay intervention when deterioration is occurring.

Isotope Studies

Cerebral scanning with radioactive isotopes may rarely be of value in those few centres where the technique is available.

SURGICAL TECHNIQUES

The emergency operations necessary for the treatment of head injury vary from the relatively simple to the quite difficult. No-one will deny that at times they present quite formidable problems.

It is essential that the occasional craniotomist should realize that when urgent operation is indicated, the patient has no chance without it. The difficulties that may arise come not from exploration, but from the problems of dealing with the lesion found. If no clot is present, a negative craniotomy is a reasonably simple and safe procedure. If clot is found, it would probably have killed the patient soon if not removed.

It is better to offer the patient some chance of survival by early operation than to delay in fright until the patient dies without or despite late operation.

Clear understanding of the nature of head injury will allow judgement in any case as to whether there is time for transport to more expert care when complications are developing on a slow time base, or whether the patient's only chance is in immediate surgery in relatively inexperienced hands.

This section sets out a ritual to be followed step by step to avoid the more obvious pitfalls that have been observed by the author.

'CRANIOTOMIES'

C onsult by telephone
R esuscitate
A irway secure
N o delay
I lluminate properly
O bserve continuously
T ools adequate
O off with all hair
M ark your incision
I nspect shaved head
E xpose adequately
S top bleeding as you meet it.

Consult by Telephone

If in doubt, ring a neurosurgeon and discuss the problem with him. Such advice is as close as your telephone, and freely available. If you report accurate observations, he can advise regarding diagnosis of complications, possibility of transfer, need for you to operate, and the most likely site for incision. You can face the patient's relatives as well as the operation with much greater confidence after such a consultation.

If in doubt, ask!

Resuscitate

You can't make an omelette without breaking eggs.

Face up to the fact that haemorrhage in some degree is inevitable, and profuse bleeding may occur.

Insert an intravenous drip before you start, have blood cross-matched ready for use, and have someone look after the transfusion for you.

Airway Secure

It is vital that the patient has an adequate airway, secure for the operation.

Suck out pharynx and larynx if necessary; insert a pharyngeal airway if this is adequate and tolerated for operations under local anaesthesia. Use an endotracheal tube (with the end in trachea and not down into bronchus) if necessary. If a general anaesthetic is given, ensure adequate strapping so that a tube does not come out when the head is inaccessible to the anaesthetist.

Support drapes away from the patient's face so that he does not rebreathe carbon dioxide.

No Delay

The earlier you operate, the easier the operation will be and the better your chance of a living patient at the end. Minutes may count.

Illuminate Properly

Arrange the lighting yourself so that it will be adequate. A headlight is the most effective way of illuminating the depths of the wound. Don't work in the dark.

Observe Continually

Make sure that someone continues routine observation of the patient throughout operation. Some factors will not be accessible; state of consciousness may be annulled by general anaesthesia, pupils obscured by the drapes. Neglect of this may lead, for example, to failure to recognize the occurrence of a major intracranial or other complication until too late during tedious suture of a large scalp laceration.

Tools Adequate

Provide yourself if possible with the minimum necessary instruments listed below. If you are stuck, a carpenter's brace and bit and a pair of pliers can achieve much.

Off with All the Hair

When you are seeking a haematoma, shave the whole head if there is any doubt as to its site. Don't be caught in the middle of an operation with an inadequate shave when you want to extend an incision. It is generally much more expeditions to shave the head yourself, in the theatre.

Remember to protect the eyes from preparation solutions and drapes by strapping them shut.

Use wet drapes so that they do not slide off the head.

Mark Your Incision

Mark the incisions likely to be needed on the scalp with pen and Bonney's blue or other dye for ink, or scratch with a scalpel after preparing *before* your drapes are put on the head. Only thus will you know exactly where your incision is. Once the head is draped, it is very easy to become disorientated with risk of completely wrong siting of your incision, inadequate exposure, and danger of damage to venous sinuses. This cannot be over-emphasized.

Mark your head before you drape!

Inspect the Shaved Head

Only after shaving may minor contusions become apparent. Search for them as the chief guide to the site of exploration.

Expose Adequately

Inspection holes are best made through small incisions, but once you find a haematoma, or a dural tear under a depressed fracture, enlarge your incision and bone opening to expose the whole lesion adequately. Don't leave half or more of a haematoma undiscovered by neglect of this.

Stop Bleeding As You Meet It

The worst mess you can get yourself into is to be paddling in a pool of blood due to haemorrhage from several layers of the wound. Stop bleeding from each layer as you open it. The methods of haemostasis are as follows:

Scalp. – Pressure with the fingertips on either side of an intended incision while the cut is made collapses the vessels against the skull.

In small wounds, a self-retraining retractor stretches the scalp and stops bleeding.

In large wounds, artery forceps applied to the galea and allowed to hang so that their weight everts the edge of scalp provide routine haemostasis.

Larger vessels such as the superficial temporal or occipital artery need to be caught separately and coagulated or ligated.

The easiest way of arresting haemorrhage from a laceration is to sew it.

Muscle. – The deep temporal arteries may need to be dealt with separately.

Bone. – Crush the diploe, or apply bone wax.

Extradural bleeding. – Place guy sutures in the dura close to bone and hang forceps on them. This approximates dura to bone and stops bleeding, especially if Gel-foam is tucked in between dura and bone. Hitch dura to pericranium for permanent control.

Dural vessels. – Diathermy, or underrun with sutures and ligate, or applying Cushing's silver clips to major vessels; diathermy or pack with gelatin sponge for minor vessels.

Cerebral veins. – Diathermy, or ligate, or pack with Gel-foam and compress lightly for ten minutes.

Small cerebral vessels. – Diathermy or pack with Gel-foam and wait.

Venous sinuses. – Sew or patch tears with crushed muscle (see under 'Depressed Fractures').

Control each layer as you cut it.

PARTICULAR OPERATIONS

Most of these are described with the lesions to which they refer: scalp injuries (Chapter 1); depressed fractures (Chapter 2); extradural haematoma (Chapter 3); subdural haematoma (Chapter 5); chronic subdural haematoma and hygroma (Chapter 11); ventriculography (Appendix 1).

Ribgraft Cranioplasty

Technique

(1) Open the scalp to expose the defect.

(2) Incise pericranium just outside the edge of the defect and strip it carefully into the hole. Thus one avoids opening the dura mater.

(3) Expose a rib and split and elevate its periosteum.

(4) Split the rib down its marrow with a chisel; borrow the outer cortical strip as a graft; leave the inner cortex as an intact thoracic cage.

(5) Take as many ribs as you need.

(6) Cut the ribs into pieces just longer than the dimension of the defect to be bridged.

(7) Chisel the skull diploe to make a shallow bed for each end of the rib.

(8) Bend the ribgraft to shorten it, and spring its end into the skull beds.

(9) If the skull is too thin to chisel, split the end of the rib into three prongs – two over, one under the skull.

(10) Make a paling-fence of rib-grafts, which need not actually touch.

Note. Don't graft until three months after the subsidence of all signs of infection.

Armamentarium

It but remains to list the desirable minimum armamentarium for the surgeon who may have to deal with head injuries (apart from the more routine surgical instruments).

Self-retraining scalp or mastoid retractors – 2 cm and 5 cm rake blades.

Narrow periosteal elevators.

Hudson brace with perforating and burring bits.

Macdonald's or McCormick's dissector.

Metal sucker (3 mm lumen) with side hole (which can be occluded by finger if necessary), to reduce power of suction on the brain.
Flat spatula malleable retractors.
Brain needles (or filling needle of a pentothal set as a substitute).
Bone nibbling forceps.
Diathermy, if possible.
A good headlight.
Gelatin sponge for haemostasis.

RECOMMENDED FURTHER READING

Kristiansen, K. (1948). 'Cerebral Angiography in the Diagnosis of Intracerebral Haematomas'. *Surgery, St. Louis* **24**, 755

Potter, J.M. (1961). *The Practical Management of Head Injuries.* London: Lloyd Luke

Vanderfield, G.K. (1961). 'Angiography in Head Injuries'. *Aust. N.Z. J. Surg.*, **30**, 292

Appendix 2

Infection

Discussion of infection in an appendix may seem inappropriate to a book on head injury, but it seemed inopportune to interrupt the general text with a consideration of post-traumatic intracranial infection.

Scalp Infection

Leave infected wounds open, or incise and drain closed infections. Search for foreign bodies or devitalized bone, and remove them. Watch for the occurrence of osteomyelitis or intracranial infection, which should rarely occur if first principles are followed.

Osteomyelitis

The full-blown picture of Pott's puffy tumour is now rarely seen, but sometimes occurs even yet. Local pain, local tenderness, oedema and erythema are leading symptoms and signs, and persistent wound discharge is most suggestive. Good quality x-rays may confirm the diagnosis.

Excise loose fragments, nibble away infected bone edges, open and drain scattered foci, and exhibit antibotics.

Meningitis

Meningitis is much more common with skull fractures compound internally into the nose, the accessory nasal sinuses, the ear or the mastoids than it is with external wounds.

The clinical picture resembles that of spontaneous meningitis, with the following variations:

(1) It may be devastatingly acute or quietly insidious.

(2) The symptoms and signs may not suggest the great severity of the infection. Especially when cerebrospinal fluid leakage from nose or ear is free, there may be little headache, little neck stiffness and surprisingly slight appearance of illness until late in the disease.

(3) Almost any organism may be found, whatever happens to be lurking in nose or ear.

(4) It can occur at any interval after injury. Diagnosis is by lumbar puncture and examination of the cerebrospinal fluid. Treatment is by antibiotics, and later repair of the responsible defect.

Cortical Thrombophlebitis

This is usually associated with meningitis, epiletic fits and localizing paresis being the leading features (in the absence of signs of space-occupying lesion).

Treatment is as for meningitis.

Venous Sinus Thrombophlebitis

Sagittal sinus thrombosis, cavernous sinus thrombosis, or lateral sinus thrombosis may all occur, each producing its typical syndrome – marasmus, facial oedema and ophthalmoplegia, and otitic hydrocephalus respectively.

Intracranial Abscess

This usually follows one of the foregoing types of infection, and may be extradural, subdural or intracerebral according to the primary focus.

To the signs of intracranial space-occupying lesion are added the general signs of suppuration, though intracerebral abscesses may be chronic and quiet.

Diagnosis is by clinical localization and exploration, or by special radiological investigation.

Treatment is by open drainage of surface abscesses, needling and aspiration of intracerebral ones.

Appendix 3

Mobilization and Rehabilitation

Only the acute phase of injury and short-term recovery period will be considered.

Mobilization

This should begin as soon as possible after the injury.

Conscious patients sit up as soon as they are able to do so comfortably, and are moved out of bed for periods according to their tolerance as soon as their state is stable or improving.

Unconscious patients have regular change of position and passive movement of all limbs from the earliest days, and follow the course for conscious patients as soon as possible.

Forced mobilization of sluggish and depressed patients, and diurnal activity for restless ones, speeds recovery.

Remedial exercises for hemiplegias or other pareses begin early.

Rehabilitation

The attitude of the doctor is of great importance. The mood of confidence and cheerful expectancy achieves much. It is unreasonable to appear to take the injury too lightly, but harmful to overstress its seriousness. Symptoms should not be callously dismissed, but explained and put into perspective.

The patient should receive instruction regarding resumption of activity at home and at employment. Too many bask in the sympathy of an over-indulgent family, lying late abed and revelling in idleness until the fateful day when they endeavour to break this habit and to do a full day's work in one major step. Fatigue from this unaccustomed stress is interpreted as inadequacy following injury, and anxiety and persistent symptoms result.

Instruction is required as to the resumption of a disciplined day consisting of return to the correct hour of rising and of meals, to establish a safe routine before work is attempted. This is the most vital step in re-training for employment.

According to the type of employment and the severity of the injury, return to work may need to be graded, as regards both type of duty and hours, with medical supervision to provide security at least.

Physiotherapist, speech therapist, occupational therapist and almoner may all be needed in the case of the disabled, together with a fully equipped rehabilitation centre, before a man returns to the dignity, the occupation and the pleasure which he should enjoy.

Appendix 4

Results

'Figures cannot lie, but liars can figure.'

C. Northcote Parkinson

One of the few available tests of any surgical discipline is the figures it produces. I have no intention of producing a mass of wearisome statistics here, but will cite only that best single index to acute care of head injury in any hospital—the mortality rates for extradural haematoma. The discipline described in this book (our daily practice) may be judged by the quality of these figures.

Recently Published Series

Hooper, R.S. (1959) 83 cases 11years 19 deaths

McKissock, W. (1960) 125 cases 19 years 34 deaths

Brisbane Hospital, Brisbane Children's Hospital, and Princess Alexandra Hospital, Brisbane.

Full Series	167 cases	11 years	26 deaths
Last 100	100 cases		10 deaths

(The Brisbane Hospital Neurosurgical Unit came into being on March 1st, 1956.)

Epilogue

This notebook has been written essentially for students of medicine, undergraduate and postgraduate, but is intended for all who care for injured patients.

It is dedicated to that group of people whose responsibility is greatest in this field—the nurses. No matter how able the doctor, the care of head injuries will never be adequate until the nurse who cares for and observes the patient understands what she is doing. She it is who prevents some complications, and diagnoses the existence of others. It but remains for the doctor to achieve differential diagnosis and treatment.

Nowhere in medicine is the nurse's responsibility greater than here, and in no other field is she so important and integral a part of the team. If perusal of these pages should direct any nurse to a clearer concept of the nature and management of head injury, their justification is complete.

Index

INDEX

INDEX

INDEX

INDEX